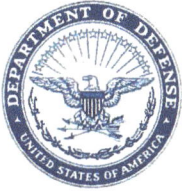

5800
Ser 100002
19 Jun 20

FINAL ENDORSEMENT

From: Chief of Naval Operations
To: File

Subj: COMMAND INVESTIGATION CONCERNING CHAIN OF COMMAND ACTIONS WITH REGARD TO COVID-19 ONBOARD USS THEODORE ROOSEVELT (CVN 71)

Ref: (a) ADM R. Burke, USN ltr 5800 Ser N09D/20U100825 of 27 May 20 (w/encl)

I reviewed reference (a), the Command Investigation, and I approve the report except as noted herein.

**Preliminary Statement**

After my review of reference (a) and the enclosures and references that inform it, I have determined that reassigning CAPT Crozier as the Commanding Officer (CO) of the USS THEODORE ROOSEVELT (CVN 71) is not in the best interest of Navy.

I make this decision fully recognizing that his email, which was leaked to the media and is the genesis of this investigation, was sent with the well-being of the crew of the USS THEODORE ROOSEVELT (CVN 71) as his top concern. Also, I am mindful that the actions of those involved must be considered with the understanding of the unprecedented nature of the challenge, the fast-pace of the crisis, and the difficulties involved with evolving guidance.

It is clear to me following this investigation, CAPT Crozier did not act according to the standards I expect of our commanding officers—to adapt in the face of adversity, exercise ingenuity and creativity in crisis, demonstrate resilience, communicate effectively up the chain of command, and to take bold and appropriate action early and often. His actions and inactions in the timeframe before sending the email fell well short of what I expect from our officers in command.

With this backdrop in mind, there are three fundamental principles that I considered as I made this decision: the nature of command at sea, the fundamental importance of the chain of command, and standards of performance in command.

Subj:   COMMAND INVESTIGATION CONCERNING CHAIN OF COMMAND ACTIONS
        WITH REGARD TO COVID-19 ONBOARD USS THEODORE ROOSEVELT
        (CVN 71)

<u>Command at Sea</u>

Title 10 of the U.S. Code requires that all commanding officers "take all necessary and proper measures "… to promote and safeguard the morale, the physical well-being, and the general welfare of the officers and enlisted persons under their command or charge." The U.S. Navy Regulations further emphasize this principle by noting in Section 0802: "The responsibility of the commanding officer for his or her command is absolute …. The authority of the commanding officer is commensurate with his or her responsibility … [and delegation of authority from him] shall in no way relieve the commanding officer of continued responsibility for the safety, well-being, and efficiency of the entire command." This Navy Regulation goes on to state: "The commanding officer … shall exercise leadership through personal example, moral responsibility and judicious attention to the welfare of persons under their control or supervision. Such leadership shall be exercised in order to achieve a positive, dominant influence on the performance of persons in the Department of the Navy." These laws and regulations underlie the nature and responsibility of command at sea, without which our Navy could not perform its critical functions. CAPT Crozier's letter and email were one means of exercising his responsibility as a commanding officer.

I believe CAPT Crozier had two critical obligations. First was to take every appropriate action possible—as quickly as possible—to safeguard the well-being of his crew in order to ensure maximum operational readiness of the THEODORE ROOSEVELT, and second, to forcefully and fearlessly communicate his observations, concerns, and recommendations up the chain of command. CAPT Crozier desired to ensure the welfare of his crew, and to accomplish this end, desired to get as much of the crew off the ship and into spaces that would allow for maximum separation. In so doing, he believed that he could ensure a "clean ship" that was ready to set sail if and when ordered to do so.

I am certain that CAPT Crozier had the best interest of the crew and the readiness of the ship he commanded in mind. However, he did not have the luxury of the best possible circumstances or time in which to meet those obligations. As explained in more detail below, CAPT Crozier did not forcefully and expeditiously execute the best *possible and available* plan, or do enough, soon enough. When faced with barriers to his primary course of action (COA), CAPT Crozier waited for others to act rather than doing what we expect of our commanding officers—to take immediate and appropriate action and to drive outcomes.

<u>Chain of Command</u>

A second bedrock principle essential to the function of the US Navy is the primacy of the chain of command. Those superior to the CO have the responsibility to clearly communicate decisions and orders down the chain of command and to consider the feedback from subordinates while the CO has the responsibility and authority to plan, decide, act and communicate up the chain of command. I expect commanding officers to fearlessly communicate up the chain of command and to have their facts straight when doing so. In the matter at hand, CAPT Crozier

2

failed to effectively communicate his concerns up the chain of command, at key moments, despite numerous opportunities to do so.

The email and the letter CAPT Crozier sent was not delivered outside the chain of command and was not intended by him to be released to the media. However, CAPT Crozier did not ensure he had all of the relevant facts and did not use available avenues to inform his chain of command prior to his sending of the letter. Specifically, he failed to pre-brief his immediate superior, Commander, Carrier Strike Group NINE (CCSG-9), who was co-located on the ship, and he excluded Commander, U.S. SEVENTH Fleet (C7F) as an addressee on his email. Importantly, his email and letter were sent hours after a decision had been made by the Government of Guam to open hotels for CAPT Crozier's crew. His email neither accelerated that decision nor had any positive impact on the outcome.

Performance in Command

CAPT Crozier's performance during this unprecedented crisis fell short in several key ways. Specifically, during the ship's transit to Guam CAPT Crozier took some steps to slow the spread of COVID-19 throughout the ship, but he did not ensure physical distancing was implemented onboard. While this is challenging on an aircraft carrier, it remained an essential preventative measure to mitigate widespread transmission.

During the critical initial 72 hour period THEODORE ROOSEVELT was inport Guam before sending his email, he did not plan for and egress sailors off the ship and onto the base fast enough. If there were obstacles to expeditious egress, he did not aggressively seek solutions. Instead, he was improperly focused on the ideal COA (hotels) and not the most likely COA (on base facilities). He narrowly focused on what he considered to be obstacles outside of his control rather than "owning the plan" by quickly and effectively implementing available options within his span of control. As well, he failed to openly communicate his concerns to senior leaders regarding the need for additional support. For instance, he did not take advantage of available opportunities to brief the entire chain of command during daily VTCs. I also hold CCSG-9 accountable for the lack of an egress plan and more rapid egress off the ship.

He also exercised questionable judgment when he released Sailors from aft quarantine onboard the ship. This allowed for increased spread of the virus onboard the ship. He placed comfort of the crew ahead of safety of the crew at a time when he should have been focused on doing everything he could to slow transmission of COVID-19 by moving Sailors ashore.

Additionally, the COA to debark the crew and place them into Guam hotels was his most desirable COA, but also the most constrained. Supporting commanders, particularly Commander Joint Region Marianas, were in direct contact with the Government of Guam on the hotels option. CAPT Crozier should have been more focused on the planning and execution of the COA to egress sailors to the facilities available on Naval Base Guam. That COA was the best path available to immediately segregate, quarantine, and isolate his crew and thus meet his first critical obligation—to safeguard the well-being of his crew in order to ensure maximum operational readiness of the THEODORE ROOSEVELT.

Finally, he did not ensure he had a full understanding of the facts before sending the email or include key members of his chain of command in the email chain. The letter did not have a positive effect on the plan in place and indeed placed undue pressure on the Governor of Guam at the time she was finalizing plans to open hotels.

**Opinions**

I endorse the Opinions found in reference (a) as follows:

Da Nang Port Visit  (Opinion 1)

I concur that the decision to execute the Da Nang, Vietnam port visit was appropriate for the reasons stated in the report. While it is likely that COVID-19 was introduced to the THEODORE ROOSEVELT as a result of this port visit, the decision-making prior to and during the visit was reasonable based on the rationale for the visit and the information known at the time.

Decisions During Transit to Guam  (Opinion 2)

The THEODORE ROOSEVELT leadership decisions during the transit were generally sound but lacked effective implementation. I note that decisions were made during a time when our knowledge of COVID-19 and its method of spread was limited and dynamic. CAPT Crozier, did, for example, enforce cleaning of ship twice daily and reminded the crew daily of the necessity to do so. Daily screening for COVID-19 symptoms were also conducted; numbers of patrons in the ships' store were limited; additional precautions were taken with respect to food preparation and meal service. The one controlling action that fell short was effective social distancing. CAPT Crozier and the rest of the leadership team directed the crew to practice social distancing, but the report reveals compliance was inconsistent. I fully recognize that *effective* social distancing is not easily accomplished at sea, though the THEODORE ROOSEVELT leadership should have worked aggressively to enforce it.

Egress of the Crew in Guam  (Opinions 4 – 9)

The CSG-9 and THEODORE ROOSEVELT leadership did not do enough to effectively plan for and execute a rapid egress of the crew in Guam consistent with the constraints and restraints present at the time. I concur with the report's conclusion that more effective planning for COAs short of off-base, fully CDC-compliant single occupancy rooms should have occurred. Specifically, CAPT Crozier and CCSG-9 should have both pushed for the most effective COA of CDC-compliant rooms, *while at the same time* doing everything possible to egress the crew onto Naval Base Guam.

However, the slow egress of the crew after arrival in Guam was influenced by numerous contributing factors. I believe each was within CAPT Crozier's span of influence to either resolve himself or seek support from his chain of command. This includes initial confusion over testing requirements prior to egress; perceived versus actual quality of berthing accommodations on Naval Base Guam; and planning requirements for the Okinawa contingency COA.

As the CO of THEODORE ROOSEVELT, CAPT Crozier should have forcefully owned the plan to quickly egress the crew given the applicable constraints and restraints, should have vigorously communicated his concerns about obstacles and resource constraints, should have insisted upon more information about ongoing efforts to secure hotel rooms, and should have pursued the interim solution of on-base berthing for his crew. However, make no mistake, the shortfalls in execution of the egress are not borne by CAPT Crozier alone. CCSG-9 as well as his staff also bear responsibility for the slow egress from the ship onto NBG.

Decision to Release Crew Members from Quarantine  (Opinion 3)

The decision to release crew members from their quarantine location in the aft portion of the ship was inappropriate. I understand CAPT Crozier's conclusion that the onboard quarantine area was crowded, uncomfortable, and may have been leading to a higher rate of infection within that area of the ship. I also understand his conclusion that numerous new positive cases onboard the ship outside of the quarantine area may have suggested that the quarantine was ineffective. CAPT Crozier's stated intent in releasing Sailors from aft quarantine was to allow for greater social distancing onboard the ship. However, he should have continued to contain the spread of the virus through quarantine while simultaneously doing everything possible to move the crew ashore. His determination that onboard quarantine was ineffective should have led to an acceleration of Sailors to ashore accommodations. It did not.

CAPT Crozier's Email and Letter  (Opinions 10, 12 – 15)

In sending the letter, CAPT Crozier's intentions were sound and I concur with the report's conclusion that he sent the letter as a "genuine plea for help." However, I also concur that the letter was unnecessary, had no positive impact on actions already underway, and should have been preceded by a clear and fulsome discussion with CAPT Crozier's immediate superior in the chain, the Commander of Carrier Strike Group NINE. While I do not believe he intended the letter to leak to the press, CAPT Crozier did intentionally omit the Commander of U.S. SEVENTH Fleet from the email. These were significant errors in judgment. Poor communication on the part of the C7F staff was a significant contributing factor in the overall poor communication throughout this chain of events. However, this does not warrant going around a member of the chain of command.

Forthright, fearless, and clear communication up and down the chain of command is essential to effective military operations, particularly when faced with a dynamic and novel threat such as COVID-19. The breakdown in communication and trust revealed in the report is troubling and certainly hampered the response to the COVID-19 outbreak.

Subj:  COMMAND INVESTIGATION CONCERNING CHAIN OF COMMAND ACTIONS
       WITH REGARD TO COVID-19 ONBOARD USS THEODORE ROOSEVELT
       (CVN 71)

In the end, the email and letter sent by CAPT Crozier were unnecessary. Although it advocated for the best COA and the one that was eventually executed, actions were already underway to acquire CDC-compliant, off-base individual hotel rooms for the crew. Before sending a direct communication three echelons up the chain of command, it is imperative that all facts are known and all other means of communication within the chain have been thoroughly exhausted. In this, CAPT Crozier fell short.

<u>Medical Department Letter</u>  (Opinion 11)

I concur that the letter signed by certain members of the THEODORE ROOSEVELT medical department was ill-conceived and inappropriate. While I do not question the desire for the medical department members to advocate for the health of the crew, it was exceedingly poor judgment to include in the letter a threat to release the letter to the public. The Senior Medical Officer (SMO) did indeed miss a leadership opportunity by signing the letter as written, even if he did not have an actual intent to release the letter. Similarly, CAPT Crozier missed a leadership opportunity when he, rather than issuing a direct order to not release the letter to the public, simply encouraged the SMO to not release it. The release of the letter, 24 hours after CAPT Crozier sent his email, was unnecessary.

**Recommendations**

(1) <u>CAPT Brett Crozier</u>. I concur that CAPT Brett Crozier will not be reassigned as the Commanding Officer of USS THEODORE ROOSEVELT (CVN 71) or to a future command, either at sea or ashore. Commander, U.S. Pacific Fleet (COMPACFLT) may consider and impose administrative measures as appropriate, based on reference (a) and based on my conclusions in this memo. CAPT Crozier's deep experience and strong history of performance should be positively considered in future assignments to key Navy positions.

(2) <u>Administrative Measures</u>. The promotion of RDML Baker is held in abeyance pending a separate review. Any decision to recommend the detachment for cause of the Senior Medical Officer (SMO) assigned to THEODORE ROOSEVELT will rest with COMPACFLT and the operational chain of command. Additionally, COMPACFLT may consider and impose administrative measures on other personnel involved in this chain of events *if warranted*, including leaders not specifically listed in Recommendation 2.

(3) <u>OPNAV Study</u>. I concur that a study of coastal state transparency as it relates to COVID-19 is useful and will help inform future port visits. I direct the Director of Navy Staff to task this project to the appropriate OPNAV staff(s).

(4) <u>Update of NTRP 4-02.10</u>. I concur with the need to update relevant health guidelines as a result of what we have learned and continue to learn about COVID-19. The Surgeon General and the Naval Warfare Development Command are directed to collaborate and update NTRP 4-02.10.

(5) <u>Cultural Workshop for THEODORE ROOSEVELT</u>.  While I do not concur that the report established a systemic or widespread lack of integrity, I do concur that operational and administrative hazards result from a breakdown in communication.  COMPACFLT may consider use of a Cultural Workshop to help the THEODORE ROOSEVELT CSG identify the root causes of the communications barriers involved in this case, and develop a learning culture that prevents similar events in the future.

(6) <u>THEODORE ROOSEVELT Medical Department Debrief</u>.  I direct the Surgeon General or his designee to debrief the THEODORE ROOSEVELT Medical Department to determine and publish best practices with regard to at-sea COVID-19 prevention, mitigation, and response.

(7) <u>THEODORE ROOSEVELT as Case Study</u>.  I direct the Vice Chief of Naval Operations to use this chain of events, the report, and my endorsement as a case study to identify, analyze, and publish lessons learned regarding the importance of clear, forthright, appropriate communication during crisis action planning and crisis response.  This study and its use must provide principles or guidelines on when and how a leader might choose to bypass a member of the chain of command.

(8) <u>CSG Commander Training</u>.  I concur with the recommendation as written and direct Director, Navy Staff to coordinate responsive action.

(9) <u>CSG Training and Certification Events</u>.  I concur with the recommendation as written and direct Commander, U.S. Fleet Forces Command and COMPACFLT to coordinate responsive action.

M. M. GILDAY

Copy to:
VCNO
COMPACFLT
COMUSFLTFORCOM
SG
JAG
DNS

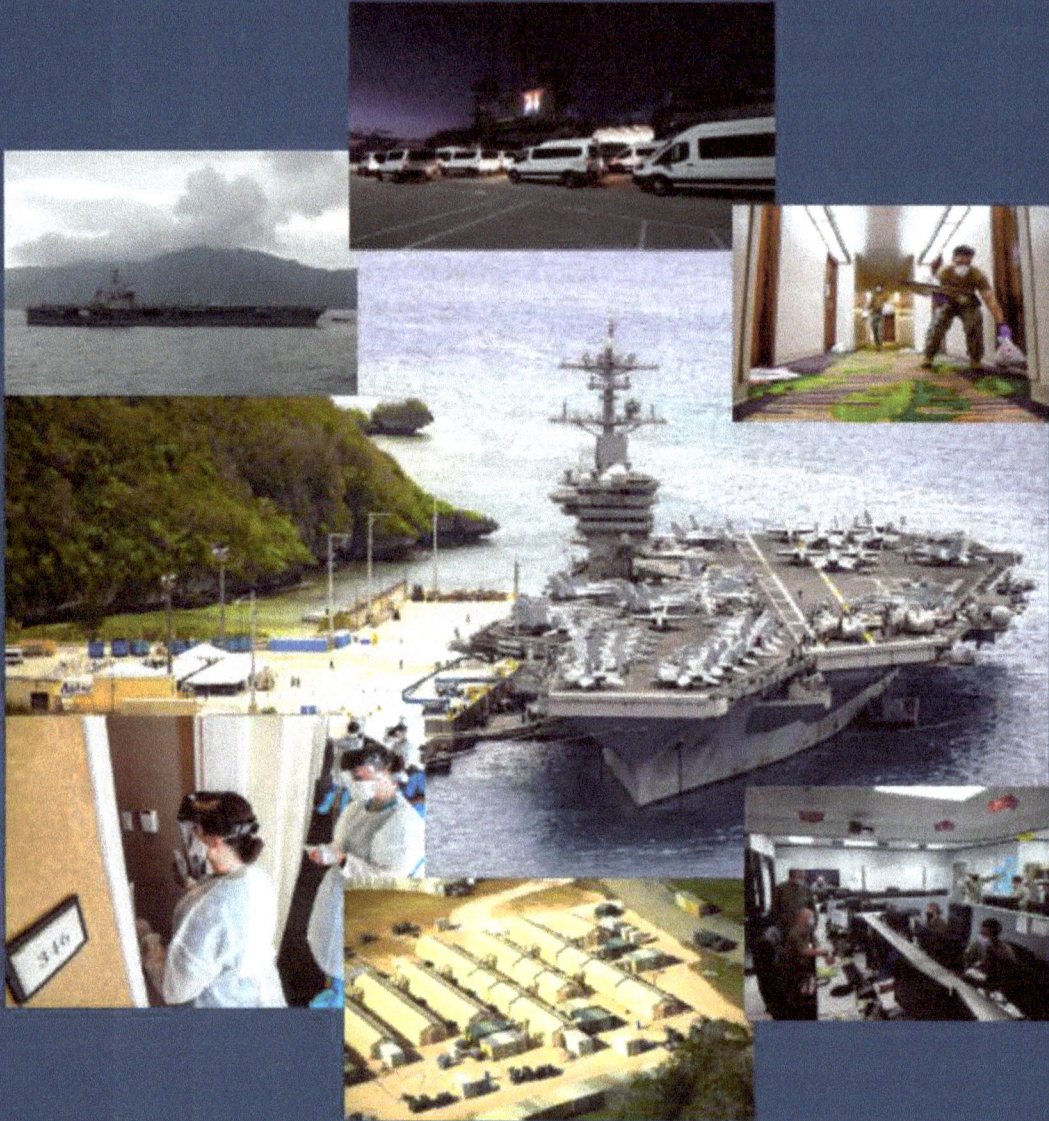

**Report of the Command Investigation Concerning**

**Chain of Command Actions**

**With Regard to COVID-19**

**Onboard USS Theodore Roosevelt (CVN 71)**

May 27, 2020

On the front cover:

Background:  USS Theodore Roosevelt (CVN-71) is moored pierside at Naval Base Guam on May 15, 2020 (US Navy Photo)

Top left:  USS Theodore Roosevelt (CVN 71) anchored off the coast of Da Nang, Vietnam, March 5, 2020 (U.S. Navy/MC3 Nicholas V. Huynh)

Top center:  Vans await to transport USS Theodore Roosevelt Sailors to quarantine and isolation facilities ashore on Guam (US Navy Photo)

Top right: US Navy Sailors assigned to local commands deliver meals to quarantined USS Theodore Roosevelt (CVN 71) Sailors in Guam hotel (US Navy Photo)

Bottom right:  Naval Base Guam Task Force Revive Command Center (US Navy Photo)

Bottom center:  Expeditionary Medical Facility established on Guam to support USS Theodore Roosevelt (CVN 71) Sailors (US Navy Photo)

Bottom left:  US Navy and USMC medical personnel conduct daily health screenings of USS Theodore Roosevelt (CVN 71) Sailors in quarantine in Guam hotel (US Navy photo)

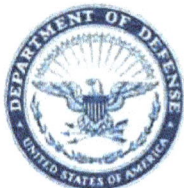

**DEPARTMENT OF THE NAVY**
VICE CHIEF OF NAVAL OPERATIONS
2000 NAVY PENTAGON
WASHINGTON DC 20350-2000

5800
Ser N09D/20U100825
27 May 20

From: Vice Chief of Naval Operations
To:   Chief of Naval Operations

Subj: COMMAND INVESTIGATION CONCERNING CHAIN OF COMMAND ACTIONS
      WITH REGARD TO COVID-19 ONBOARD USS THEODORE ROOSEVELT
      (CVN 71)

Ref:  (a) Your ltr 5800 Ser N00J of 30 Apr 20

Encl: (1) Final Report

1.  Reference (a) directed me to inquire into the communications, decisions and actions that took place within the Navy chain of command related to the following matters:

    a.  Planning and execution of the Da Nang, Vietnam port visit.

    b.  Transit of USS THEODORE ROOSEVELT (CVN 71) to Guam, including air movements during transit and planning for the ship's arrival and provisions for the crew.

    c.  Actions following arrival of USS THEODORE ROOSEVELT (CVN 71) to Guam, including movement of the crew to on-base and off-base lodging.

    d.  Preparation and email delivery of the former commanding officer's letter dated 30 March 2020, further handling of that email, and response to the email and letter by the chain of command. I was directed to include in my report transcripts or summaries of public statements made by Department of the Navy officials related to the relief of the former commanding officer, without rendering opinions or recommendations on the relief or the rationale behind it.

2.  Enclosure (1) is my final report into these matters.

R. P. BURKE

**Table of Contents**

Preliminary Statement

Executive Summary

Chapter 1 - Introduction

Chapter 2 - Planning and Execution of Port Visit to Da Nang, Vietnam

Chapter 3 - Actions during Transit to and Arrival in Guam

Chapter 4 – Development of and Response to Commanding Officer's Letter

Chapter 5 – Opinions and Recommendations

Appendix A – Appointing Letters

Appendix B – Investigation Team

Appendix C – Timeline of Events

Appendix D – Findings of Fact

Appendix E – Preliminary Inquiry

Appendix F – Analysis of Binnacle List

Appendix G – Master List of Citations

Appendix H – Supporting Documents

Appendix I – Transcript of Public Statements

Appendix J – Classified Supporting Documents

**Preliminary Statement**

This command investigation inquired into the communications, decisions, and actions that took place within the Navy chain of command related to the Coronavirus Disease 2019 (COVID-19) outbreak aboard USS Theodore Roosevelt (CVN 71) (TR). It expanded upon the work done for the preliminary inquiry (located at Appendix E) to investigate more deeply into four key areas, and to ensure more complete documentation of events. The Navy has already implemented the institutional and procedural changes recommended by the preliminary inquiry.

In order not to risk the possible reintroduction or spread of COVID-19, the command investigation team did not travel to visit the TR. Instead, the command investigation team relied primarily upon video-conferences, telephone calls, and electronic means to collect evidence, with the full support of all command levels involved.

All times in this report are Guam Local Times (Chamorro Standard Time), unless otherwise noted (e.g., for events that occurred in the continental United States or Pearl Harbor, Hawaii).

The command investigation team did not encounter any difficulties during the course of their investigation, and received the full cooperation of every witness who was interviewed.

The command investigation team took great care to understand the perspective of a leadership team dealing with an unprecedented challenge. The learning curve for COVID-19 has been steep, and the investigation team made every effort to consider the findings relative to guidance existing at the time of the events described in this report.

With respect to the specific matters the investigation was tasked to examine, the team concluded:

1. The decision process and calculus for approving TR's port visit to Da Nang was appropriate. The planning for the Da Nang port visit was done with careful, methodical and thorough consideration of the status of the COVID-19 outbreak in Vietnam at the time. The risk analysis was advised by experts and data from the U.S. Centers for Disease Control and Prevention (CDC), the World Health Organization (WHO), and after consultation with the government of Vietnam to better understand their methods and measures for COVID-19 control. At that time, based upon the data available, it reasonably appeared to be safer in Vietnam than many domestic U.S. Navy fleet concentration areas. The visit was executed with sensible precautions, based on the world's understanding of

COVID-19 at the time.

2. During the transit of TR from Vietnam to its mission operating area, and then to Guam, with 39 Sailors in quarantine, no significant additional precautions were taken for the remainder of the crew until fifteen days after leaving Da Nang. Sailors had reported to the Medical Department as early as three to four days after leaving Da Nang, but the symptoms were not able to be correlated with COVID-19, even with assistance from embarked Biological Defense Research Directorate (BDRD) teams and their limited COVID-19 surveillance testing capability. After the first Sailors began to test positive for COVID-19 on March 24th, few additional precautions were directed for those not isolated or quarantined, despite the known potential for asymptomatic transmission.

3. After arrival in Guam, available off-ship berthing was not aggressively used, due to the TR leadership insisting on fully CDC compliant quarantine quarters. Although the off-ship makeshift berthing was not perfect, it provided vastly improved ability to socially distance crewmembers. Miscommunication over testing requirements also contributed to significant delays in egressing the crew, initially. The TR and Commander, Carrier Strike Group Nine (CCSG-9) leadership spent the majority of their efforts finding flaws with the Commander, U.S. 7th Fleet (C7F) intended way ahead, while offering no practicable solutions and neglecting to supervise and coordinate the crew's egress to temporary off-ship quarantine facilities. Finally, due to an erroneous conclusion that the shipboard quarantining efforts were causing more Sailors to be infected, the ship ceased its quarantine efforts on March 29th, with over 4,000 Sailors still aboard. This was done without consultation or notification to higher headquarters, and apparently was not discovered by higher headquarters leadership until the preliminary inquiry. The combination of these actions likely contributed to increased spread of the infection to more TR Sailors.

4. As to the former TR CO's email and attached letter, he was present at C7F staff meetings where discussions took place regarding the efforts in progress to secure longer-term, CDC compliant quarters for his crew. He, therefore, knew or should have known of the actions that were already underway up echelon, but was dissatisfied with the interim quarters. Rather than lead his team to work with the shore establishment to improve upon them, he elected to send his email and attached letter. When it was later leaked to the media, it complicated the Navy's negotiation with the Government of Guam for use of hotel rooms in Guam. The identity of the person leaking the email remains unknown.

It is clear that TR received exceptional support and resources from all levels of the chain of command. It is also clear that the dynamically evolving situation required robust and rapid communications from Echelon I down to the command level. The findings of this investigation identified that typical leadership style differences, combined with the complexity of the problem, and an absence of lessons learned from which to draw, all contributed to some communications breakdowns up and down the chain of command. However, these communications breakdowns were largely inconsequential.

At the core of this set of seemingly coincidental and perhaps even understandable minor errors was an unpredictable virus spreading exponentially among the crew, a sense of moral responsibility to protect the health of the Sailors, and lack of a clear and effective command element, from the strike group and down. These factors led to a command team becoming biased by groupthink, emotion and a loss of perspective as to the *real* risk at hand. Their actions did not align with the fleet commander's efforts to help get the crew off of TR rapidly, and they were seemingly unaware of the efforts being worked on their behalf by multiple entities. The commanding officer's email and letter changed nothing – all of the actions requested were in play before he sent the email.

It is difficult to comprehend how the entire command team, driven by an overwhelming concern for the crew's safety, took little to no action within their own span of control to improve the crew's safety. The leadership team was missing in action when it came to leveraging available temporary facilities, organizing and then leading a quick and effective egress from the ship. Not recognizing their missed leadership opportunity, it became necessary, in their minds, to further disregard good order and discipline by "jumping the chain" [of command] with an urgent plea.

After 40 plus days to reflect on their actions since arrival on Guam, many of the principal members of the ship and strike group leadership team maintain that their actions to protect the crew were proper, and that the actions requested would not have occurred without the former commanding officer's email and letter.

Setting aside the combination of factors that led to delays in getting the TR crew ashore, there are two significant actions that were inconsistent with existing guidance at the time and had significant consequences for the spread of the virus throughout the ship:

1. The lack of measures taken for the majority of the crew after March 24th.

2. The release of Sailors from quarantine aboard the ship on March 29th.

Following the COVID-19 outbreak, the level of support to TR from multiple individuals and organizations, including the Governor of Guam and her staff, Commander, Joint Region Marianas (CJRM) and his staff, Commanding Officer, Naval Base Guam (CO, NBG) and his staff, III Marine Expeditionary Force (III MEF) element, and Commander, Task Force (CTF) 75 was both extraordinary and unprecedented.  TR's Sailors have helped our Navy and nation learn much in our response to the COVID-19 crisis.

To date, the Navy has had over 50 ships with COVID outbreaks and each of them has responded with vigor to control and manage the spread of the virus in order to remain mission ready.  The Navy took the valuable lessons learned from TR and rapidly revised and improved upon fleet-wide COVID prevention, mitigation, recovery, and pre-deployment guidance, providing risk-informed direction to afloat units regarding how to better manage the virus.

As the world continues to learn every day about COVID-19, it is becoming clear that the young and healthy demographic that the U.S. Navy enjoys with its Sailors means that we can confidently fight through any future outbreaks on our warships.  That said, if we have the operational flexibility, we will not ask that of our Sailors or their families.

## Executive Summary

Introduction

On March 24, 2020, three Sailors aboard USS Theodore Roosevelt (CVN 71) (TR) tested positive for COVID-19 while the ship was underway in the western Pacific Ocean. TR was a little more than two months into a five and one-half month long deployment, and at the time of the discovery, was transiting the 2,500 miles between her last port call in Da Nang, Vietnam, and her next one in Guam. The events that transpired before TR's port call in Vietnam, during the transit to and following her arrival in Guam are the subject of this investigation.

As TR began her deployment, the world was starting to understand an illness that began in China and whose spread quickly challenged nations around the globe. The chronology of the outbreak aboard TR in March, 2020 parallels that of the illness's spread throughout the world. As governments, including our own, have learned about COVID-19's transmission, symptoms and nature, the United States Navy has learned from TR's experience regarding how to prevent, mitigate and recover from an outbreak in the unique environment of a deployed naval vessel.

Port Visit in Vietnam

On January 17, 2020, the TR and Carrier Strike Group Nine (CSG-9) departed San Diego for deployment. The same week, C7F began tracking COVID-19's spread in the Pacific. By early February, as TR and one of the destroyers in the strike group, USS Pinckney (DDG 91), pulled in for their first port visit to Guam, WHO had declared the COVID-19 outbreak a "Public Health Emergency of International Concern." WHO confirmed the virus was a pandemic on March 11th.[1]

The same week in March 2020, TR pulled into Da Nang, Vietnam for a visit intended to fulfill an agreement between the U.S. and Vietnam. The port visit, only the second by a U.S. aircraft carrier to the country since the Vietnam War, was timed to commemorate the 25th anniversary of bilateral relations between the two countries.[2] At the time of TR's arrival in Da Nang, there were no State Department, Defense Department or CDC travel restrictions for U.S. citizens to Vietnam.[3]

---

[1] "WHO Timeline - COVID-19." World Health Organization, www.who.int/news-room/detail/27-04-2020-who-timeline---covid-19
[2] CPF Statement dtd 17 May 20
[3] INDOPACOM J07 Country Health Risk to Force for COVID-19 dtd 4 Mar 20

On March 8[4], the Vietnamese Government notified CSG-9 that Sailors on liberty from TR and the USS Bunker Hill (CG 52) (BKH) may have been exposed to COVID-19 at a hotel in Da Nang, as two tourists who stayed at that hotel tested positive for the virus.[4] TR and BKH curtailed the port visit and got underway shortly thereafter with 39 Sailors in quarantine aboard the carrier.[5]

Transit from Vietnam to Guam

On March 9[th], TR got underway from anchorage in Da Nang Bay, Vietnam, and resumed normal operations in the C7F area of operations. An outbreak of norovirus in February led the ship's crew to clean common touch areas, which continued throughout the visit to Da Nang.[6] Although the CO limited self-service in the galley,[7] other ship's services continued as usual, such as barbershops, ship's store, chapel and gyms.[8]

From the time the ship left Da Nang on March 9[th] until March 23[rd], seven Carrier Onboard Delivery (COD) flights originating out of Clark Air Force Base in the Philippines brought a total of 29 passengers and COD detachment personnel to the carrier,[9] all of whom screened negative for COVID-19 symptoms upon their arrival.[10] Later, four of those personnel tested positive for the virus, however analysis of the time of their positive results indicates that they were likely not the source of the introduction of the virus. Having arrived via COD on March 3[rd], the prospective TR Executive Officer (XO) conducted a planned turnover with his relief on March 11[th].[11]

As TR sailed to Guam, the island's government declared a public health emergency on March 14[th], even though no COVID-19 cases had yet been identified on the island.[12] By March 17[th], all 50 U.S. states had confirmed cases of the virus[13] and by March 20[th], Guam had 12 confirmed cases of COVID-19.[14]

On March 22[nd], after a 14-day quarantine period, all 39 Sailors potentially exposed to

---

[4] Email - AMB to Vietnam - Status of Sailors from Vietnam dtd 8 Mar 20
[5] TR XO Statement dtd 16 May 20
[6] TR XO Statement dtd 16 May 20, TR SMO Statement dtd 17 May 20
[7] Email - TR CO to TR SMO - Follow Up dtd 9 Mar 20; TR SUPPO Statement dtd 18 May 20; TR XO Statement dtd 16 May 20
[8] TR SMO Statement dtd 17 May 20 "The barber shops, ship's store, chapel, and gyms remained open and there was no discussion about closing them down at this time, nor was this the recommendation put out by higher headquarters."
[9] COD Completed Travel Log/Manifest, TR SMO Statement dtd 17 May 20
[10] Crozier, B. CAPT Statement dtd 15 May 20; TR XO Statement dtd 16 May 20; CVW-11 CAG Statement dtd 19 May 20
[11] Email - TR XO - TR Investigation dtd 7 May 20
[12] Government of Guam Executive Order 2020-03
[13] CORONAVIRUS: DOD RESPONSE TIMELINE (15 May 20) https://www.defense.gov/Explore/Spotlight/Coronavirus/DOD-Response-Timeline/
[14] Email - NBG CO to TR CO - TR PVST dtd 20 Mar 20

COVID-19 in Da Nang remained asymptomatic, tested negative for COVID-19 and were released from quarantine.[15] However, on March 23[rd], two air wing (CVW-11) Sailors aboard TR began showing symptoms of the virus.[16] Those two, and an additional Sailor from the ship's nuclear reactor department, tested positive for COVID-19 on March 24[th].[17] None of these three Sailors were among the 39 who had been potentially exposed to the virus in Da Nang and subsequently placed in quarantine.

By the next day, four Sailors were positive for COVID-19, and TR moved them ashore to Naval Hospital Guam via helicopter.[18] On March 25[th], discussions began at the staff level among CSG-9, TR, CJRM, and C7F regarding the potential need for 4,000-plus people to move off the ship.

During the transit from Vietnam, based on Preventative Medicine theory, TR and CSG-9 informed C7F on March 25[th] that the quickest way to return TR to sea would be "to house all personnel in individual isolation for two weeks."[19] CSG-9 requested permission from C7F to discuss the feasibility of contracting hotel rooms with JRM to ensure they were not surprising the Government of Guam.[20] C7F COS stated that "this is a big ask" and did not express confidence that such a course of action had a high probability of success, and that C7F wanted to explore other options.[21] The courses of action that relied on housing 4,000 Sailors ashore on Guam were deemed the most constrained and least likely. Accordingly, C7F focused their attention predominantly on the COA to transport Sailors to Okinawa.

Using every available resource on the remote Pacific Island, CO, NBG offered berthing arrangements that met many but not all of the requested parameters. The discussion of CDC compliant, individual rooms was not brought up again by CSG-9 or TR until the C7F staff meeting on March 29[th], although CJRM continued to work for hotel rooms on Guam in parallel on March 28[th], 29[th] and 30[th].[22]

As concern elevated up TR's operational and administrative chains of command, on March 26[th] (CONUS), the Commander, U.S. Pacific Fleet (CPF) and the Chief of Naval Operations (CNO) exchanged emails noting that the plan was to test the entire TR crew

---

[15] C7F COS Statement dtd 21 May 20; Crozier, B. CAPT Statement dtd 15 May 20; TR XO Statement dtd 16 May 20; TR SMO Statement dtd 17 May 20
[16] Email - TR SMO to CCSG-9 - COVID-19 Update dtd 24 Mar 20
[17] Email (SIPR) - CCSG-9 COS to C7F COS - Hotel Option dtd 25 Mar 20; Email - TR SMO to CCSG-9 - COVID-19 Update dtd 24 Mar 20
[18] "Sailors tested positive on USS Theodore Roosevelt, extent of exposure unclear" Pacific Daily News (26 Mar 20)
https://www.guampdn.com/story/news/local/2020/03/26/sailors-tested-positive-uss-roosevelt-extent-exposure-unclear/5084652002/#
[19] Email - TR SMO to CCSG-9 - COVID-19 Update dtd 24 Mar 20
[20] Email - TR SMO to CCSG-9 - COVID-19 Update dtd 24 Mar 20
[21] Email - TR SMO to CCSG-9 - COVID-19 Update dtd 24 Mar 20
[22] Email – CJRM to VCNO EA - RE: Follow-up RFI dtd 6 Apr 20

for COVID-19.[23]  These notes would later be construed by some to mean that testing would be required prior to the crew leaving the ship and setting foot on Naval Base Guam, causing confusion and delaying crew egress.

On March 27th, TR arrived in Guam and moored at the pier[24] with 36 COVID-19 positive Sailors aboard the carrier.[25]

Arrival Guam

A number of factors converged to delay TR Sailors from occupying all available facilities on Guam.  Providing food for the number of TR Sailors ashore in isolation and quarantine was a challenge.[26]  As this capacity continued to ramp up, and the number of Sailors ashore increased, contracted food delivery lagged initially, and TR Sailors expressed their concerns on social media.  This was relayed to the TR CO and TR XO.[27]  Additionally, the ship's leaders were concerned that the temporary open-bay facilities did not meet CDC guidelines.  In reaction to the social media posts and out of concern for the living conditions ashore, the TR CO prevented Sailors from leaving the ship until a guarantee of sufficient meal service was available.[28]

A lack of clarity about the quality and type of facilities ashore, as well as lack of clarity over testing requirements before leaving the ship, also contributed to delays in disembarking the TR crew.  Prior to TR's arrival, CO, NBG, C7F and CCSG-9 agreed on a plan to transport Sailors who were COVID-19 positive and Reactor Department Sailors (key backup watchstanders) to rooms ashore immediately.  On TR's first day in port, 264 Sailors moved ashore.[29]  However, there was no plan at that time to move ashore the large number of Sailors now quarantined on the ship, nor was there clarity on any requirement to test crew members prior to going ashore to NBG.  Prior to the hotels becoming available, the testing requirement for Sailors going ashore was not well understood by the TR CO, XO, and Senior Medical Officer (SMO).[30]  During interviews, the C7F COS stated that 100 percent testing was not required and that message was clearly communicated, however e-mails from him and C7F prior to the ship's arrival

---

[23] Email (SIPR) - CPF to CNO and INDOPACOM - TR Recovery and Disposition Plan dtd 26 Mar 20
[24] Facebook Post - Family and Friends of the Rough Riders, Crozier, B. CAPT (27 Mar 20)
https://www.facebook.com/USSTheodoreRoosevelt/photos/a.489137065779/10156700551025780/?type=3&theater
[25] Email (SIPR) - C7F - C7F COVID daily CDRs update (26 Mar) dtd 27 Mar 20
[26] NBG CO Statement dtd 18 May 20; TR XO Statement dtd 16 May 20
[27] Crozier, B. CAPT Statement dtd 15 May 20; TR XO Statement dtd 16 May 20; TR PAO Interview Summary dtd 23 May 20
[28] Crozier, B. CAPT Statement dtd 15 May 20
[29] Email - CJRM - Follow-Up Summary of Interview dtd 8 May 20
[30] Crozier, B. CAPT Statement dtd 15 May 20; TR XO Statement dtd 16 May 20; TR SMO Statement dtd 17 May 20

implied testing was required.[31]  Similarly, several emails from higher headquarters, to include the Office of the Chief of Naval Operations (OPNAV) and CPF, implied the same.[32]  This was being driven by a belief at the time that 100 percent testing of the crew could be quickly completed, and a relatively modest number of TR crew members could be left on Guam to recover, allowing the ship to return to sea.  This belief also reflected the complete lack of understanding that existed at the time of the limitations of the available testing means.  Combined with imprecise communications, confusion ensued.  For example, during interviews, the TR CO stated that testing was required, the XO stated that 100 percent testing was not being conducted, and the SMO stated that he was confused over testing requirements but did not agree with 100 percent testing.[33]  This contributed to the delay in getting potentially non-infected crewmembers off the ship into available facilities on Guam,[34] that, although not ideal and not meeting the strict CDC guidance of single room and single bathroom per individual, did offer better protection from infection than the ship's berthing compartments and messing facilities.

C7F believed that the TR CO and CCSG-9 were resisting sending the crew ashore because available facilities were not fully CDC compliant.[35]

On March 28th, C7F tasked CCSG-9 and TR to develop plans to airlift crew members to Okinawa.  C7F prioritized other COAs over the Guam hotel room option at this point due to the conditions under which the Navy had obtained permission to bring TR into the naval base – the Navy had agreed that Sailors would remain on the naval base, and that the Navy would not ask for help from the Government of Guam, as Guam was itself in a state of public health emergency.  C7F was aware and although CJRM is not under his authority C7F asked him to work directly with the Governor of Guam to entertain the hotel option.

The TR CO, unaware of C7F's work with III MEF to obtain 5,000 CDC compliant rooms on Okinawa, contacted an acquaintance, Commander, Fleet Activities Okinawa (CFAO), on the same island.  CFAO was also unaware of the III MEF work, and told the TR CO that 5,000 rooms were not available for TR Sailors.[36]  The CSG-9 COS and CVW-11 CAG both stated that they believed the 5,000 beds never existed.  As a result of this lack of clarity in the Okinawa plan, further friction developed between the TR CO,

[31] C7F COS Statement dtd 21 May 20; Email (SIPR) - C7F COS to CSG-9 COS - Triage and Procedure dtd 27 Mar 20
[32] Email (SIPR) - C7F to CPF - Evening Update and COVID 29 Mar dtd 29 Mar 20
[33] C7F COS Statement dtd 16 May 20; Crozier, B. CAPT Statement dtd 15 May 20; TR XO Statement dtd 16 May 20; TR SMO Statement dtd 17 May 20
[34] C7F COS Statement dtd 21 May 20; Crozier, B. CAPT Statement dtd 15 May 20;TR XO Statement dtd 16 May 20
[35] C7F COS Statement dtd 16 May 20
[36] Crozier, B. CAPT Statement dtd 15 May 20; TR XO Statement dtd 16 May 20; Email - CAPT Crozier to Commander, Fleet Activities Okinawa – Subj: New Normal dtd 29 Mar 20, 1818

XO, CVW-11 CAG, CSG-9 COS and the C7F staff.[37]  The TR CO made no effort to confirm the status of the Okinawa rooms with anyone in his chain of command.

By the ship's fourth day in Guam, the TR CO and Warfare Commanders began to believe there were no plans to move 4,000 crew off the ship into isolation and quarantine in CDC compliant facilities.[38]  In the meantime, the commander of the Carrier Air Group (CVW-11 CAG) embarked on TR led a collective effort with the Warfare Commanders and TR senior leadership to develop courses of action to improve the situation for TR's crew.  The CSG-9 leaders wanted to minimize the number of Sailors exposed to COVID-19 and regain warfighting readiness as soon as possible.[39]  CSG-9 leaders grew increasingly frustrated with the proposed way ahead and wanted CCSG-9 to address what they believed was a crisis by demanding the crew be offloaded as soon as possible to hotel rooms in Guam.[40]  At the same time, CCSG-9 believed the use of hotels in Guam was not currently an option for TR because of political concerns.[41]  Unsatisfied with the response he had received so far from his efforts to ask CCSG-9 to champion the hotel room COA with C7F, on March 30th, the TR CO sent an email to "Fellow Naval Aviators" with a memo requesting "all available resources to find NAVADMIN and CDC compliant quarantine rooms for my entire crew as soon as possible."[42]  The San Francisco Chronicle published this memo online the next day.[43]  At the time of this writing, the individual(s) responsible for releasing the letter to the SF Chronicle remains unknown.

Additionally, although the TR CO stated that he was not fully aware of the status of efforts underway to open Guam hotels to TR Sailors, he should have known by his presence at C7F briefs and through discussions with CCSG-9.[44]  The TR CO also stated that he did not anticipate the potentially negative implications his letter could have had to ongoing negotiations that same day between CJRM and the Governor of Guam.[45]

---

[37] Crozier, B. CAPT Statement dtd 15 May 20; TR XO Statement dtd 16 May 20; CVW-11 CAG Statement dtd 19 May 20; CSG-9 COS Statement dtd 18 May 20
[38] Crozier, B. CAPT Statement dtd 15 May 20; TR SMO Statement dtd 17 May 20; CVW-11 CAG Statement dtd 19 May 20
[39] CVW-11 CAG Statement dtd 19 May 20
[40] CSG-9 COS Statement dtd 18 May 2020
[41] CCSG-9 Statement dtd 18 May 20;  Email (SIPR) – CSG-9 COS to C7F COS – (U) HOTEL OPTION dtd 25 Mar 20
[42] TR CO Email and Ltr - Request for Assistance in Response to COVID-19 Pandemic dtd 30 Mar 20
[43] "Exclusive: Captain of aircraft carrier with growing coronavirus outbreak pleads for help from Navy" SF Chronicle (31 Mar 20) https://www.sfchronicle.com/bayarea/article/Exclusive-Captain-of-aircraft-carrier-with-15167883.php, accessed May 8, 2020
[44] Crozier, B. CAPT Statement dtd 15 May 20; Email - CJRM - Follow-Up Summary of Interview dtd 8 May 20; CCSG-9 Statement dtd 15 May 20; C7F Statement dtd 18 May 20
[45] Crozier, B. CAPT Statement dtd 15 May 20; Email - CJRM - Follow-Up Summary of Interview dtd 8 May 20

Actions after Publication of Memo

CCSG-9 did not understand the rationale for the TR CO's memo, as he knew at the time, and thought the TR CO knew, efforts to pursue all requested courses of action were already underway. According to CCSG-9, the memo's publication created tension between with the Navy and the Government of Guam, potentially complicating negotiations for the ship's crew to occupy hotels on the island.[46]

On April 1st, Commander Naval Air Force, U.S. Pacific Fleet (CNAP) called the TR CO in Guam to provide mentorship and counsel and to learn why he felt the need to write the email and memo. TR CO relayed that his relationship with C7F and CCSG-9 were healthy, with good communications in both directions, and plenty of communication opportunities. The TR CO also noted C7F was particularly engaged, holding multiple video-teleconferences each day regarding the situation on the TR. In response to CNAP's question, the TR CO stated his rationale for sending the memo was that he did not feel the shore establishment's response was moving fast enough.[47]

The TR SMO also sent a letter off the ship on March 31st, outlining areas of concern of the medical staff aboard, and a threat to release the letter to the media if immediate actions were not taken. This letter did not outline specific requests but did relay a sense of urgency. It calculated that at least 50 Sailors would die from COVID-19 based on data received and analysis conducted on the potential mortality rate.[48] The SMO emailed the medical letter to eight people initially, addressed to the Surgeon General of the Navy and copying seven others. The SMO then emailed the letter to over 160 additional email addresses, primarily individuals within the Navy Medical community and outside his operational and administrative chains of command.[49]

However, no new actions were taken as a result of either the TR SMO's or the TR CO's email and letter, as the actions they desired were already in motion.[50] In fact, CJRM had begun staff level discussions with the Governor's office about the possibility of securing hotel rooms on March 28th, and spoke with the Governor herself later that day, receiving a positive response.[51] This allowed Navy to finalize staffing up to Commander, United States Indo-Pacific Command (INDOPACOM), where it was decided that CPF would call the Governor of Guam to formally request assistance on

---

[46] CCSG-9 Statement dtd 15 May 20; Email - CJRM - Follow-Up Summary of Interview dtd 8 May 20
[47] CNAP Statement dtd 13 May 20
[48] Email – SMO to Surgeon General - Medical Dept Letter dtd 30Mar20
[49] Email – SMO - FWD: Medical Dept Letter dtd 30Mar20
[50] Email – CJRM to VCNO EA - RE: Follow-up RFI dtd 6 Apr 20; C7F Statement dtd 18 May 20
[51] Email – CJRM to VCNO EA - RE: Follow-up RFI dtd 6 Apr 20; Email - CJRM - Follow-Up Summary of Interview dtd 8 May 20; C7F Statement dtd 18 May 20

March 31st.[52]  The positive response also allowed Navy to begin formal negotiations with GHRA regarding the number of hotels and the conditions for their utilization.[53]  CJRM was extremely sensitive to the publicly stated Navy position to not over burden Guam resources and as a result, information on those efforts was not widely known outside of the principals on the various staffs.[54]  However, according to C7F and CCSG-9, TR CO was aware of these efforts.[55]

CNO ordered a preliminary inquiry into the events surrounding the disembarkation of Sailors from TR in Guam, in response to cases of COVID-19 on April 2, 2020.[56]  While this preliminary inquiry was pending, the A-SN at the time decided to relieve the TR CO and announced his decision in a press conference with the CNO, stating that "at [his] direction, the CO of [TR] . . . was relieved by [CCSG-9]."[57]

The A-SN subsequently traveled to Guam where he spoke with members of the TR crew via the public address system (1MC).  Those remarks were recorded by members of the crew and released to the press by means of a written transcript followed by the actual audio recording.[58]  Following his visit to TR and subsequent calls for his resignation, including from House Armed Services Committee Chairman, Adam Smith (D-WA),[59] the A-SN offered his resignation to the Secretary of Defense on April 7th, 2020,[60] and his resignation was accepted that same day.[61]  The preliminary inquiry ordered by CNO was also completed on April 7th, and had been submitted to CNO prior to the A-SN's resignation.

Current Status of TR Crew

Although most TR Sailors with the virus displayed mild symptoms, 45 Sailors were admitted to Naval Hospital Guam for treatment for COVID-19.  Of these Sailors, six required oxygen support and one was placed on a ventilator for respiratory failure.  The majority were admitted for close observation and did not require additional intervention.[62]  One Sailor died due to complications attributed to COVID-19.  A

---

[52] C7F Statement dtd 18 May 20; CPF Statement dtd 17 May 20
[53] Email - CJRM - Follow-Up Summary of Interview dtd 8 May 20
[54] Email - CJRM - Follow-Up Summary of Interview dtd 8 May 20
[55] C7F Statement dtd 18 May 20; CCSG-9 Statement dtd 15 May 20
[56] CNO Ltr Ser 5800 dtd 2 Apr 20
[57] Transcript:  DON Press Briefing with Acting Secretary of the Navy Thomas B. Modly and CNO Admiral Gilday dtd 2 Apr 20
[58] How a Ship's Coronavirus Outbreak Became a Moral Crisis for the Military, NY Times, (6 Apr 20) https://www.nytimes.com/2020/04/06/us/politics/coronavirus-navy-secretary-roosevelt-crozier.html (containing audio recording of A-SN remarks)
[59] Press Release: "Smith Calls for Modly's Removal After Mishandling U.S.S. Theodore Roosevelt COVID-19 Outbreak" dtd 6 Apr 20
[60] A-SN Resignation Letter of 7 Apr 20
[61] SECDEF Ltr of 7 Apr 20
[62] CO NHG Statement dtd 18 May 20

separate line of duty investigation into the circumstances of his death has been completed.

As of the writing of this report, a total of 1,248 TR crewmembers were infected with the COVID-19 virus, 1,546 TR Sailors remain in Guam, and 498 are positive, continuing quarantine and testing, with one currently hospitalized. TR is at sea today, conducting operations. Over 100 other ships are also at sea, operating around the world, without known COVID cases aboard.

## Summary of Opinions

*The following 18 key opinions were derived from this investigation into the COVID-19 outbreak aboard TR:*

1. **Based upon the pre-event risk analysis, the decision to execute the Da Nang port visit was appropriate. The visit was executed with sensible precautions, based on the world's understanding of COVID-19 at the time.**

2. **The former TR CO initially responded appropriately by quarantining 39 Sailors following the Da Nang port visit. However, after three Sailors tested positive for COVID-19 aboard TR on March 24, 2020, the former TR CO failed to put adequate additional measures in place for the rest of the crew to further slow the spread of COVID-19 throughout the ship.**

3. **The TR SMO's recommendation and the resulting release by the former TR CO of crewmembers in quarantine from the aft portion of the ship on March 29, 2020 likely resulted in infection to a larger portion of the crew.**

4. **The embarked CSG-9 Warfare Commanders (WCs) (TR CO, CVW-11 CAG, DESRON Commodore) and the TR SMO displayed an abundance of concern for the safety of the crew as their primary focus, yet they were unable to develop COAs prior to or even by four days after arrival in Guam that provided for the short-term safety of the crew. Instead, they focused efforts on the most constrained and least executable COA (at the time), while taking insufficient parallel steps that would have resulted in more immediate segregation, quarantine and isolation of the crew. As a result, efforts to move the crew off the ship were uncoordinated, unsupervised and slow. The extended time Sailors remained on the ship, while no longer segregated, likely increased the number of infections.**

5. **CCSG-9, the embarked CSG-9 WCs, and the former TR CO and TR SMO did not demonstrate effective leadership when they initially took few actions to overcome obstacles to aggressively utilize the approximately 2,300 beds that were made available by Naval Base Guam, likely resulting in infection to a larger portion of the crew.**

6. **C7F's early focus on the Okinawa option over the Guam hotel option resulted in the TR Strike Group key Captains (CSG-9 COS, former TR CO, TR XO, TR SMO and CVW-11 CAG) believing that C7F did not feel their same sense of urgency for providing proper long term quarantine and isolation quarters. This led these Captains to distrust the C7F staff and hampered their ability to deal with the crisis with the resources that were available, or develop alternate courses of action other than the request for 4,000 CDC compliant rooms, which at the time was the most constrained and least likely COA.**

18

7. *The former TR CO did not demonstrate forceful backup, effective communication or adequately communicate with his Immediate Superior in Command (CCSG-9, embarked in TR) in that he did not discuss his concern with the lack urgency he perceived from C7F and CCSG-9 on the Guam Hotel option being pursued, prior to sending his letter.*

8. *CCSG-9 did not provide effective leadership to the former TR CO and the embarked CSG-9 WCs in that he did not effectively address and correct a growing, divisive and counterproductive narrative among his senior officers regarding distrust of C7F or any course of action that did not fit their immediate sense of urgency. Additionally, he did not direct decisive action to ensure prompt execution of the egress of the TR crew. Finally, it is not clear that he effectively advocated for TR's needs to higher headquarters or provided clear feedback to his team when those needs could not meet TR leadership's timeline.*

9. *The TR SMO developed a flawed, worst-case crew casualty narrative that the CVW-11 CAG reinforced and frequently amplified at Warfare Commander Boards, and that had an impact on the mindset of the former TR CO and TR XO. The TR SMO fostered distrust of HHQ actions, and put his leadership in an untenable situation.*

10. *The TR CO sent his email and letter as a genuine plea for help from CPF and CNAP. Each leader received and acted upon it as such, responding via phone and email, respectively, within minutes of receipt, with CNAP also ensuring C7F and CJRM were made aware of the request. Further, CPF considered the matter of sending the letter closed after his conversation with both CCSG-9 and TR CO.*

11. *When asked to sign a letter that contained a flawed, worst-case crew casualty narrative as well as an ultimatum concerning an intent to submit the letter to the public, the TR SMO missed a leadership opportunity to correct subordinates. Instead, he signed the letter, and transmitted it outside the chain of command, essentially endorsing the effort to undermine Navy leadership.*

12. *The former TR CO intended for his email to be a "red flare" to accelerate needed support and ensure attention to what he believed to be insufficient courses of action. The former TR CO wrote his email to break down communication barriers on plans, resources and support, and did not intend for it to be released to the public. However, he did not personally inform his Immediate Superior in Command, CCSG-9, of the letter and instead transmitted information of a very sensitive nature about a capital warship on an unclassified network.*

13. *The exclusion of C7F on the former TR CO's email, as well as the lack of advanced coordination by the former TR CO with CCSG-9 and others, bypassed the operational chain of command and demonstrated poor judgment.*

14. *The former TR CO's email and the attached letter of March 30, 2020 were unnecessary, and had no positive impact on actions already being aggressively pursued by higher headquarters (CJRM, C7F, and CPF).*

15. *Release of the former TR CO's letter to the San Francisco Chronicle complicated the Navy's negotiations with the Government of Guam for use of hotel rooms in Guam.*

16. *Detailed patient history analysis of the 29 personnel received aboard TR via COD following the Da Nang port visit concluded that CODs were not the likely source for the COVID-19 outbreak. Although the pre-event risk analysis for the Da Nang port visit was assessed as sufficiently thorough and the decision to the execute the port visit was appropriate at the time, the Da Nang port visit was found to be the most likely source of the outbreak on TR.*

17. *Detailed analysis of TR sick call logs revealed that COVID-19 was likely present, yet undetected, as early as March 11, 2020.*

18. *The use of personal protective equipment (PPE) and employment of tactics, techniques, and procedures (TTP) by the TR Medical Department were likely effective, as there was only one COVID-19 infection among TR Medical Department personnel.*

## Chapter 1 – Introduction

On March 24, 2020, three Sailors aboard USS Theodore Roosevelt (CVN 71) (TR) tested positive for COVID-19 while the ship was underway in the western Pacific Ocean. TR was transiting the 2,500 miles between her last port call in Da Nang, Vietnam, and her next one in Guam. By the time TR arrived in Apra Harbor, Guam on March 27th, 36 Sailors had tested positive for COVID-19, and many more were being isolated to prevent further infections due to their close contact with the ill Sailors. Three days later, on March 30th, TR's Commanding Officer (CO) emailed senior officers, attaching a letter detailing his concerns about the developing situation and potential impact to TR Sailors. The San Francisco Chronicle obtained, and on March 31st, published, the TR CO's letter. On April 2nd, in Washington, D.C., the CNO directed the Vice Chief of Naval Operations (VCNO) to conduct a preliminary inquiry into the events surrounding the disembarkation of Sailors from the TR in Guam. On April 3rd (Guam date), the A-SN directed CCSG-9 to relieve the TR CO of command. On April 7th (Washington, D.C. date), the VCNO submitted the completed preliminary inquiry to the CNO, and later that day, the A-SN resigned.

## Scope of Investigation

In a memorandum dated April 29, 2020, the A-SN directed the CNO to convene a command investigation into the communications, decisions, and actions that took place within the Navy chain of command related to an outbreak of the Coronavirus Disease 2019 (COVID-19) aboard TR. On April 30, 2020, and in response to A-SN's memorandum, CNO appointed the VCNO as the investigating officer to complete an in-depth investigation to inform CNO's review of the status of the former commanding officer of the TR, and to enable full consideration of the following matters:

1. Planning and execution of the Da Nang, Vietnam port visit.

2. Transit of TR to Guam, including air movements during transit and planning for the ship's arrival and provisions for the crew.

3. Actions following arrival of TR in Guam, including movement of the crew to on-base and off-base lodging.

4. Preparation and email delivery of the former commanding officer's letter dated March 30, 2020, further handling of that email, and response to the email and letter by the chain of command.

CNO directed VCNO to report findings of fact, opinions, and recommendations in writing to CNO no later than May 27, 2020.

The command investigation followed and expanded upon a preliminary inquiry VCNO completed at the direction of CNO that focused on communications involving the ship's health care professionals, commanding officer, and administrative and operational chains of command. The preliminary inquiry also outlined events related to the ship's port visit in Da Nang, Vietnam, and subsequent arrival in Guam.

This report does not evaluate the actions of non-Department of the Navy agencies.

Methodology

The VCNO assembled an investigation team comprised of subject matter experts in safety investigations, naval supply systems, carrier aviation, intelligence, human factors, law, medicine, and other unrestricted line communities. Appendix B contains a roster of team members.

The investigation team reviewed documents, interviewed witnesses, and conducted field observations and met daily to relay and synchronize findings and determine the need for additional information.

Members divided into three teams to focus on 1) the port visit to Da Nang; 2) actions during TR transit to and arrival in Guam; and 3) development of and response to TR's Commanding Officer letter dated March 30, 2020.

Report Organization

The report is organized in chapters that analyze the major elements of the appointing order. Chapter 2 examines the planning and execution of the ship's port visit to Da Nang, Vietnam from March 5 through 9, 2020. Chapter 3 examines actions of various organizations and individuals during TR's transit to and arrival in Guam. Chapter 4 examines the development of and response to TR's Commanding Officer's letter of March 30, 2020. Chapter 5 provides detailed Opinions and Recommendations.

## Background

USS Theodore Roosevelt (CVN 71) (TR) is America's fourth Nimitz-class aircraft carrier with a crew of about 4,800 Sailors who support and conduct air operations at sea.[63] The TR is part of CSG-9, which is comprised of a total of about 7,000 Sailors, and includes, in addition to the aircraft carrier, an air wing, a cruiser and five destroyers. Prior to deploying for the western Pacific on January 17, 2020, CSG-9 deployed in support of Operations Inherent Resolve and Freedom's Sentinel, as well as maritime security cooperation efforts in U.S. 5th and 7th Fleet areas of operations from October 2017 to May 2018.  In March 2020, CSG-9 was deployed and operating under the command of U.S. 7th Fleet, having reported a change in operational control ("chopped") from U.S. 3rd Fleet during the transit across the Pacific from San Diego.

The aircraft carrier is a lethal, high-end, survivable platform capable of full spectrum warfare and provides a wide range of options to the U.S. government, from demonstrating presence, to deterring adversaries, to reassuring our allies and partners. Because carriers operate in international waters, their aircraft do not need to secure landing rights on foreign soil.  These ships also engage in sustained operations in support of other forces.  When deployed as a strike group, the ships and aircraft may take on a variety of roles, all of which involve the attainment and maintenance of sea control, such as protecting commercial and military shipping, protecting a Marine Amphibious Force, or establishing naval presence, all in support of our National Defense Strategy.

COVID-19 is a newly identified viral respiratory disease caused by the SARS-CoV-2 virus.  It is responsible for a large pneumonia outbreak in Hubei Province, China resulting in the exportation of cases globally.  On March 11, 2020, WHO declared the global outbreak of COVID-19 a Pandemic (global spread of a new disease) due to virus sustainment on more than six continents, exceeding 120,000 infected persons worldwide.  Public health measures continue to be implemented and executed in hopes of viral containment such as social distancing, teleworking and minimizing social gatherings to consist of no more than 10 people.  State emergencies were declared throughout the United States to enforce these measures and many Governors issued statewide Stay at Home orders.  On March 29, 2020, President Trump extended the social distancing order until April 30, 2020.[64]

---

[63] OPNAV Instruction 5450.337B Missions, Functions, and Tasks of Commander, United States Pacific Fleet dtd 21 Jan 16
[64] Remarks by President Trump, Vice President Pence, and Members of the Coronavirus Task Force in Press Briefing (30 Mar 20) https://www.whitehouse.gov/briefings-statements/remarks-president-trump-vice-president-pence-members-coronavirus-task-force-press-briefing-14/

## Relevant Chains of Command

This investigation spans multiple chains of command, from the ship to U.S. Pacific Fleet. The Navy's command structure is more complex than other military services in that there are two chains of command: operational and administrative. They sometimes overlap, and depending on assignment, a unit can be part of both or can switch between two different operational chains of command as it transits the world's oceans. The operational chain of command is responsible for carrying out specific missions such as operations and exercises. The administrative chain of command takes care of personnel, education, training, repairs and supply chains to get ships, squadrons, and strike groups ready for those missions.[65] CSG-9 administrative and operational chains of command are outlined below and depicted in Figure 1.

## Administrative Chain of Command

CSG-9's administrative chain of command runs through CNAP. CNAP is administratively responsible to the four-star Commander, U.S. Pacific Fleet (CPF) for ensuring the readiness of all assigned naval aviation units, including aircraft carriers, deploying in the Pacific Fleet. The three-star admiral who serves as CNAP is also the Commander, Naval Air Forces (CNAF), the Type Commander (TYCOM) responsible to CPF for the readiness of all naval aviation units worldwide. This report focuses on the role of CNAP in relation to CSG-9.

## Operational Chain of Command

When operating in or near home port in San Diego, California, CSG-9 is part of U.S. 3rd Fleet, which leads naval forces in the near Pacific and provides the realistic, relevant training necessary before forces deploy away from U.S. shores. U.S. 7th Fleet, the U.S. Navy's largest numbered fleet, conducts forward-deployed naval operations in support of U.S. national interests in the Indo-Pacific area of operations. The three-star admirals commanding U.S. 3rd Fleet (C3F) and U.S. 7th Fleet (C7F) coordinate to plan and execute missions based on their complementary strengths to promote ongoing peace, security, and stability throughout the entire Pacific theater of operations. This report covers a timeframe in which CSG-9 was predominantly within the C7F operational chain of command.

---

[65] OPNAVINST 5400.45 Standard Navy Distribution List Administrative Organization of the Operating Forces of the U.S. Navy dtd 1 Apr 20

CSG-9 itself consists of the following ships and subordinate commands:

1. Carrier Strike Group 9, commanded by a rear admiral (O7) who serves as the strike group's composite warfare commander and will be referred to throughout as the Commander, Carrier Strike Group 9 (CCSG-9)

2. USS Theodore Roosevelt (CVN 71), commanded by a captain (O6)

3. USS Bunker Hill (CG 52), a Ticonderoga-class guided missile cruiser, commanded by a captain (O6)

4. Destroyer Squadron 23, commanded by a captain (O6), and comprising five Arleigh Burke-class destroyers, each commanded by a commander (O5):

   - USS Russell (DDG 59)

   - USS Paul Hamilton (DDG 60)

   - USS Pinckney (DDG 91)

   - USS Kidd (DDG 100)

   - USS Rafael Peralta (DDG 115)

5. Carrier Air Wing (CVW) 11, commanded by a captain (O6) (CVW-11 CAG), and comprising nine other units, all but one commanded by a commander (O5):

   - Four Strike Fighter Squadrons (VFA): VFA-31, VFA-87, VFA-146 and VFA-154

   - Carrier Airborne Early Warning Squadron (VAW) 115

   - Electronic Attack Squadron (VAQ) 142

   - Helicopter Maritime Strike Squadron (HSM) 75

   - Helicopter Sea Combat Squadron (HSC) 8

   - Fleet Logistic Support Squadron (VRC) 30 Detachment 3 (O4 Officer in Charge)

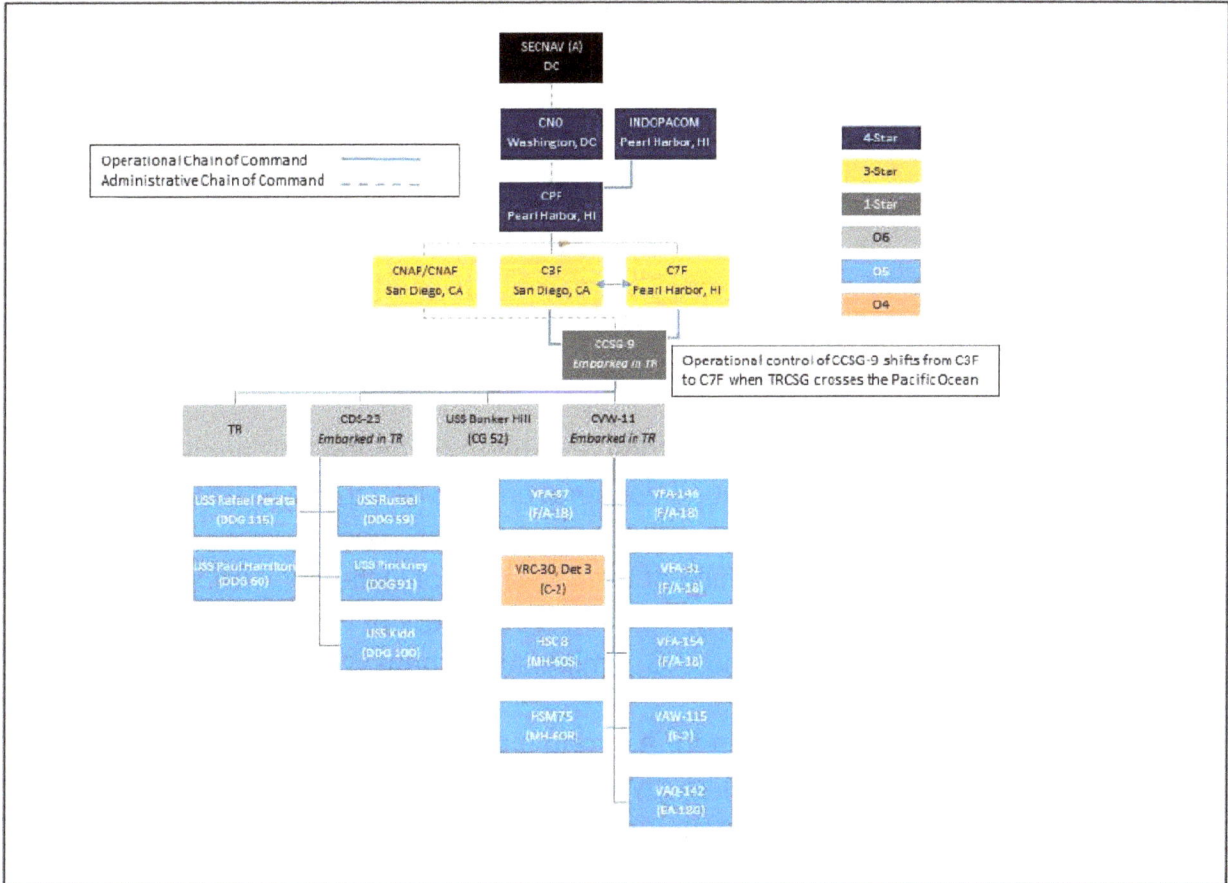

Figure 1. Theodore Roosevelt Carrier Strike Group Chains of Command

## Chapter 2 – Planning and Execution of USS Theodore Roosevelt (CVN 71)  Port Visit to Da Nang, Vietnam

Preparation for Da Nang, Vietnam Port Visit

The CSG-9 port visit in Da Nang, Vietnam was scheduled for March 5-9, 2020 with both the USS Theodore Roosevelt and the USS Bunker Hill scheduled to participate.[66]  This historic port visit fulfilled an agreement between the two nations' top leaders and was only the second visit by a U.S. aircraft carrier to the country since the Vietnam War.[67]

The visit also marked a significant milestone commemorating the 25[th] anniversary of bilateral relations highlighting continued cooperation between the U.S. and Vietnam.[68] A visit of such significance draws interest from and requires coordination among United States Department of State, The Office of the Secretary of Defense, INDOPACOM, Commander, U.S. Pacific Fleet (CPF), Vietnamese Ministry of Foreign Affairs, Vietnamese Ministry of Defense, and U.S. Embassy Vietnam.[69]

In order to demonstrate U.S. support for a strong, prosperous, and independent Vietnam and to strengthen relations, many interpersonal interactions were scheduled, including distinguished visitor engagements, special events, and tours, highlights for Sailors as well as for the people of Vietnam.  Beyond celebrating and strengthening relations, the Strike Group deployment and port visit served many other purposes. Naval presence in the Pacific region is routine and has helped maintain peace for more than 70 years.  Operating in the region supports regional security, stability, and prosperity.  Operating in accordance with international laws, rules, standards, and norms across the region enables us to reassure our allies and partners, and keeps global trade flowing.

As CSG-9 continued planning and preparing for the port visit to Vietnam, on December 31, 2019, Wuhan Municipal Health Commission, China, reported a cluster of cases of pneumonia in Wuhan, Hubei Province which was eventually identified as novel coronavirus.  On January 13, 2020, officials confirmed a case of COVID-19 in Thailand, the first recorded case outside of China.[70]

---

[66] CPF Statement dtd 17 May 20
[67] TRNOTE 5050 TR and CVW-11 Liberty Plan dtd 22 Feb 20; CCSG-9 Statement dtd 15 May 20
[68] CPF Statement dtd 17 May 20
[69] TR AAR For 5-9 March Vietnam PVST dtd 17 Mar 20
[70] WHO Timeline - COVID-19." *World Health Organization*, World Health Organization, www.who.int/news-room/detail/27-04-2020-who-timeline---covid-19

On January 17[th], CSG-9 departed San Diego for deployment.[71]  On January 20[th], in an email to TR leadership, TR XO reminded them that six weeks remained until the Da Nang port visit.  Compared to the March 2018 USS Carl Vinson (CVN 70) Da Nang port visit After Action Report, the TR XO believed they still had a lot of work to do, considering they had not done much internal planning, to ensure a successful visit.[72]

C7F began COVID-19 planning and socialization at the end of January and on January 25[th], they sent slides to all CTF surgeons.[73]

On February 2[nd], two cases of norovirus were documented aboard TR.[74]  Noroviruses are very contagious and are the most common cause of gastroenteritis in the U.S. Symptoms include diarrhea, vomiting, nausea, and stomach cramping.[75]  Within 24 hours, ship-wide precautions were established including: stopping self-service on the main galley line and requiring the culinary specialist to serve the food in order to prevent the spread of germs, thorough cleaning periods, termed "bleach-a-palooza," and general messaging regarding handwashing and personal hygiene.  These swift and sweeping actions led to eradication of the norovirus on TR prior to arrival Da Nang.[76]

On February 7[th], TR and USS Pinckney arrived in Guam for a scheduled port visit.[77]  Two weeks later, the C7F flagship, USS Blue Ridge (LCC 19),[78] and ships from the America Expeditionary Strike Group (AESG), USS America (LHA 6), and USS Green Bay (LPD) had port visits in Thailand.[79]  On January 30[th], the WHO Director General declared the COVID-19 outbreak a "Public Health Emergency of International Concern."[80]  Following this declaration, INDOPACOM directed a formal response to the pandemic[81] and the C7F Fleet Surgeon provided CPF a COVID-19 Concept of Operations (CONOPs).[82]  On February 15[th], C7F published Tasking Order (TASKORD) 20-057 for force health protection against COVID-19 and a week later, on February 22[nd], TR released the liberty plan for Da Nang[83] with no mention of COVID-19 or

[71] CNAP Statement dtd 13 May 20
[72] Email - XO to TR Leadership - Vietnam Planning dtd 20 Jan 20
[73] C7F Surgeon Statement dtd 23 May 20
[74] Email: CSG-9 – Response to RFI dtd 17 May 20
[75] NTRP 4-02.10 dtd Sep 14
[76] TR PA Statement dtd 12 May 20
[77] USS Theodore Roosevelt and USS Pinckney Arrive in Guam for Scheduled Port Visit USS Theodore Roosevelt PAO (7 Feb 20) https://www.c7f.navy.mil/Media/News/Display/Article/2077194/uss-theodore-roosevelt-and-uss-pinckney-arrive-in-guam-for-scheduled-port-visit/
[78] USS Blue Ridge, 7th Fleet staff arrive in Thailand USS Blue Ridge Public Affairs (22 Feb 20) https://www.cpf.navy.mil/news.aspx/130560
[79] USS America, Green Bay arrive in Thailand for Cobra Gold Zline, V. MC3 (23 Feb 20) https://www.cpf.navy.mil/news.aspx/130559
[80] WHO Director-General's statement on IHR Emergency Committee on Novel Coronavirus (2019-nCoV) https://www.who.int/dg/speeches/detail/who-director-general-s-statement-on-ihr-emergency-committee-on-novel-coronavirus-(2019-ncov)
[81] Naval Message (SIPR): USINDOPACOM, Response To Novel Coronavirus EXORD DTG 040649Z FEB 20
[82] Naval Message (SIPR): USINDOPACOM, Response To Novel Coronavirus EXORD DTG 040649Z FEB 20
[83] TRNOTE 5050 TR and CVW-11 Liberty Plan dtd 22 Feb 20

coronavirus. On February 25[th], Vietnam suspended entry for all travelers from COVID-19 affected areas.

On February 23[rd], C7F published Fragmentary Order (FRAGORD) 001 to TASKORD 20-057, revising disease surveillance and screening requirements due to updated country risk. On February 24[th], the CDC posted information for travelers regarding apparent community transmission in Singapore, Thailand, and Vietnam, and recommended travelers reconsider cruise ship voyages in Asia.[84] At this point, 16 confirmed cases had been reported in Vietnam, all located 30 miles outside of Hanoi, and more than 450 miles from Da Nang. On February 25[th], Vietnam suspended entry for all travelers from COVID-19 affected areas.

Senior medical experts at all levels in the chain of command (TR SMO, C7F and CPF Fleet Surgeons) were in close coordination throughout the port visit planning process. As part of their discussions, they noted that the number of COVID-19 cases reported in Vietnam for the two weeks prior to the visit remained constant, causing them to question the validity of the reported data. To resolve this concern, the CPF Surgeon conducted a phone call with the CDC director on-site in Vietnam, who relayed strong confidence in the reported data because of first-hand observations of Vietnam's transparency in executing COVID testing, prevention and mitigation actions.[85] CPF had a discussion with the U.S. CDC Country Director in Vietnam (USCDCVN). USCDCVN informed CPF that there was "no direct/indirect evidence to suggest an undetected coronavirus outbreak within the country." He also stated "that he feels the visit is truly low risk and that the Vietnamese response to the COVID outbreak is truly impressive."[86] This assessment resulted in medical staff concurrence that the health risk for the port visit was low when conducted in accordance with the February 27[th], 2020 CPF COVID-19 EXORD. The medical team, however, recommended to and gained approval from C7F[87] to significantly curtail exchange events ashore, reducing the time and numbers of TR Sailors ashore.[88]

On February 29[th], Vietnamese media reported the CDC removed Vietnam from its list of areas experiencing widespread or sustained community transmission of COVID-19. The CDC and the U.S. Department of Health and Human Services "lauded Vietnam for achieving positive results in tackling COVID-19 epidemic." As of February 29[th], the number of confirmed cases in Vietnam remained at 16. WHO continued to advise

---

[84] Update Public Health Response to the Coronavirus Disease 2019 outbreak - United States (24 Feb 20) https://www.cdc.gov/mmwr/volumes/69/wr/mm6908e1.htm
[85] Email - CPF Surgeon to TR SMO and C7F Surgeon - Discussion with CDC Director dtd 26 Feb 20
[86] Email - CPF Surgeon to TR SMO and C7F Surgeon - Discussion with CDC Director dtd 26 Feb 20
[87] Email - C7F to VCNO EA - COMREL Rel and Med Visits in Da Nang dtd 15 Apr 20
[88] Email - C7F to VCNO EA - COMREL Rel and Med Visits in Da Nang dtd 15 Apr 20

against the application of travel or trade restrictions to countries experiencing COVID-19 outbreaks.[89]  On February 25th, the last person (#16) left a Vietnamese hospital after testing negative for COVID-19, leaving no active cases of COVID-19 in the country.[90]

In preparation for the growing pandemic, on February 29th, C7F requested support from Navy Environmental and Preventive Medicine Unit (NEPMU) teams, with equipment from Navy Medical Research Center (NMRC) for forward deployable preventative medicine units to mitigate the potential outbreak of COVID-19 aboard America Expeditionary Strike Group (AMA ESG) and CSG-9 ships.  Based on this assessment C7F concluded that COBRA GOLD was a higher risk than Vietnam and the medical support was deployed to the Blue Ridge and AMA ESG.[91]

Reviews were completed daily up until the day prior to the port visit.  Having considered this latest information and issued preventative guidance regarding COVID-19, CPF recommended to Commander, INDOPACOM on March 4th that the port visit continue as planned.[92]

CDC personnel in Da Nang worked with the Vietnam Country Team and provided information to INDOPACOM.  CDC and Country Team continued to support TR's port visit to Da Nang, also assessing it as low risk to the ships' crews.

The TR SMO emailed TR's crew a COVID-19 screening plan, which required all personnel to be screened for COVID-19 symptoms prior to boarding the ship, and again seven days after getting underway.  At this point, it was not widely known that asymptomatic carriers could spread the virus.

The Da Nang Medical Treatment Plan called for inbound aircraft flights to be screened at the Department Level.  This screening consisted of monitoring for flu-like illness, and if present, sending them for an immediate medical evaluation vice waiting for routine sick call.  TR leadership (TR XO, CMC, and SMO) made initial preparations for potential quarantine quarters aboard ship by identifying appropriate berthing compartments and discussing the general plan for execution.[93]

Before the port visit, the ship had outlined three quarantine plan options:

1.  Distinguished Visitor (DV) Row

---

[89] WHO Recommendations for International Traffic (29FEB20) https://www.who.int/news-room/articles-detail/updated-who-recommendations-for-international-traffic-in-relation-to-covid-19-outbreak
[90] Nguyen, Trang H D, and Danh C Vu.  "Summary of the COVID-19 outbreak in Vietnam - Lessons and suggestions." *Travel medicine and infectious disease*, 101651.  2 Apr. 2020, doi:10.1016/j.tmaid.2020.101651
[91] C7F Surgeon Statement dtd 23 May 20
[92] Email (SIPR) - CPF to USINDOPACOM - DECISION: Theater Posture Operations dtd 4 Mar 20
[93] TR XO Statement dtd 16 May 20; TR CMC Statement dtd 17 May 20; TR SMO Statement dtd 17 May 20

- Six rooms (two-person officer staterooms, used for guests, cots for additional patients)

2. Berthing

- Chief Petty Officer overflow berthing (open-bay berthing)

- Admin Department male berthing (open-bay berthing, currently occupied)

- Medical Quiet Room (four bunks with an attached bathroom)

3. Brig

- Up to 20 bunks (between two cells, open-bay berthing)

They also planned for use of specific heads, food delivery, laundry delivery, trash and medical checks.[94] Although not listed in the presentation, quality of life items such as exercise equipment and computer and phone availability were also planned.[95]

The TR crew liberty brief stated that COVID-19 is a respiratory virus spread mainly person to person when an infected person coughs or sneezes.[96] The brief noted that 82 percent of COVID-19 cases are classified as a mild illness, and that CDC did not recommend those feeling well wear face masks, which was correct for that timeframe.[97] The brief directed Sailors to report to a Medical Detachment at Fleet Landing prior to boarding the ship if they experienced fever, body aches, cough, or felt sick.[98] The liberty brief also contained information on gun shops and weapons, tattoo/piercing establishments, local pharmacies, designated liberty/leave area, hotel/lodging, unofficial tours, and other items.[99]

The Community Relations Project (COMREL) CONOPs, dated March 1st, showed the scope of precautions being taken in Vietnam. For example, the CONOPs noted that the Agent Orange Victims Center, one of the sites for which a COMREL was planned, was "closed to students due to COVID-19, so Sailors will conduct community service events such as maintenance, repairs, and improvements to center."[100]

---

[94] TR SMO PowerPoint - Quarantine Plan and COVID Mitigation Measures "En Route to 'Nam"
[95] TR CMC Statement dtd 17 May 20, TR XO Statement dtd 16 May 20; CVW-11 CAG Statement dtd 19 May 20
[96] TR Da Nang Port Visit Overview Brief dtd Mar 20
[97] TR Da Nang Port Visit Overview Brief dtd Mar 20
[98] TR Da Nang Port Visit Overview Brief dtd Mar 20
[99] TR Da Nang Port Visit Crew Brief dtd Mar 20
[100] COMREL CONOPs dtd 1 Mar 20

On March 2nd, health officials announced the first two U.S. deaths tied to coronavirus that occurred among patients in a suburb of Seattle, Washington, as well as the first known U.S. cases of the virus among health care workers who had treated coronavirus patients.[101]  Some individuals infected with COVID-19 have no symptoms, but can still transmit the virus—a phenomenon that changed the face of the virus and presented a new obstacle to researchers trying to curb transmission of the virus."[102]  It was reported that for the majority of cases, patients show mild symptoms.  According to researchers from the University of Hong Kong, most mild cases of the virus were indistinguishable from a common cold, and that other symptoms could include mild fatigue and a low fever.[103]

On March 2nd, TR's Prospective Executive Officer (PXO) arrived via COD.[104]

On March 3rd, TR facilitated two distinguished visitor (DV) daylight-only visits to the ship.[105]  The first visit consisted of 17 Vietnamese nationals nominated by the Government of Vietnam (GVN) while the second consisted of 14 U.S. country team members who planned the port visit.  Tour routes were designed to minimize internal access to the ship and visitor use of handrails and other touch surfaces.[106]

The next day, CPF forwarded the final port visit decision recommendation to INDOPACOM, who approved it.[107]  The day's INDOPACOM Country Health Risk to Force for COVID-19 indicated that Vietnam's current risk status was "yellow," signifying moderate risk where COVID-19 cases occur in the community without known contacts or exposures and/or with small outbreak clusters, swiftly handled by public health interventions that limit disease transmission.  The risk level was projected, in seven days, to be "green," signifying low risk countries with no reported cases of COVID-19, or countries that have cases that were imported from another country, or countries that have isolated transmission exclusively attributed to travel, household contacts or healthcare settings.  The CDC and State Department reported Level 1 for Vietnam, which recommended practicing usual precautions.

It is unusual for CPF and INDOPACOM to be involved in the decision regarding a port

---

[101] America Has Suffered Its First Coronavirus Deaths-and First Infections of Health Care Workers." *Advisory Board- Daily Briefing*, www.advisory.com/daily-briefing/2020/03/02/corona-deaths
[102] "America Has Suffered Its First Coronavirus Deaths-and First Infections of Health Care Workers." *Advisory Board- Daily Briefing*, www.advisory.com/daily-briefing/2020/03/02/corona-deaths
[103] "Some Coronavirus Patients Don't Show Symptoms. Here's Why That's a Problem." *Advisory Board Daily Briefing*, www.advisory.com/daily-briefing/2020/03/02/asymptomatic-coronavirus
[104] TR XO Statement dtd 16 May 20
[105] TR Da Nang Port Visit Overview Brief dtd Mar 20
[106] TR PAO Interview Summary dtd 23 May 20
[107] Email (SIPR) - CPF to USINDOPACOM - DECISION: Theater Posture Operations dtd 4 Mar 20

visit.[108]  However, because COVID-19 had begun spreading beyond China, there was heightened interest and scrutiny from upper echelons to ensure appropriate risk analysis and mitigation measures were implemented to keep the crew safe and execute as much of the port visit mission as possible.[109]

## TR and USS Bunker Hill Port Visit to Da Nang

TR anchored in Da Nang Bay and USS Bunker Hill (BKH) moored pier side in Da Nang on March 5th.[110]  At the time of TR's arrival in Da Nang, there were no State Department, Defense Department, or CDC travel restrictions for U.S. citizens to Vietnam.  Vietnam restricted travel only from China, Republic of Korea, Iran, and Italy before the day of arrival.[111]

When the TR and BKH arrived in Da Nang, a Vietnamese delegation formally received the United States Ambassador to Vietnam, Ambassador Kritenbrink, CPF, CCSG-9, and the Commanding Officers of USS Theodore Roosevelt and USS Bunker Hill on the pier.[112]  The group posed for a photo prior to a press conference attended by more than 100 reporters.  The Vietnamese Ministry of Foreign Affairs moderated the 60-minute press conference.  Ambassador Kritenbrink, CPF and CCSG-9 participated with two Vietnamese representatives - Mr. Huynh Duc Truong, Director of Da Nang Department of Foreign Affairs and Mr. Ho Ky Minh, Vice Chairman of Da Nang People's Committee. Reuters, Channel News Asia and Da Nang Newspaper, were among the media outlets called upon for questions focused on the visit's historical significance, the U.S.-Vietnam bilateral relationship, and Naval operations in the South China Sea.

Ambassador Kritenbrink, CPF, Consulate General Damour (Ho Chi Min City) and CCSG-9 attended office calls with the Chairman of the Da Nang People's Committee and Vietnamese Commander of Navy Region 3.

On March 5th, although all reported COVID-19 cases in Vietnam were reported as clear, CSG-9 and local authorities continued to take precautions to prevent the spread of the virus.  Some events were cancelled, and liberty restrictions were enforced.[113]  TR and BKH Sailors were limited to visiting only Embassy-vetted locations and hotels.  Both TR and BKH cleaned the ships with bleach and disinfectant daily.  High sea-states limited

---

[108] CPF Statement dtd 17 May 20
[109] CPF Statement dtd 17 May 20
[110] CPF Statement dtd 17 May 20;
[111] INDOPACOM J07 Country Health Risk to Force for COVID-19 dtd 4 Mar 20
[112] TR AAR For 5-9 March Vietnam PVST dtd 17 Mar 20
[113] CCSG-9 Statement dtd 15 May 20; XO, TR CMC Statement dtd 17 May 20; Crozier, B. CAPT Statement dtd 15 May 20

the ability of TR Sailors to attend liberty events, resulting in the cancellation of two planned sporting events, many tours and community relations events, often the highlights of a port visit for a ship's crew. However, more than 100 other strike group personnel and U.S. Country Team members fulfilled all the other Community Relations Project obligations, which included interacting with residents at the Vocational Charity Center, Dorothea's Project Legacy Charity Center (attended by Ambassador Kritenbrink, CPF and CCSG-9), Agent Orange Victims Center, Hoa Mai Orphanage and Dong A University. Local media covered these events and interviewed strike group personnel.

CPF hosted a formal reception for 500 guests on March 6th. Originally scheduled to be held aboard TR, the event was moved to Da Nang Golden Bay Hotel due to concerns with safely transferring guests to and from the carrier because of an increased sea state. CPF, AMB Kritenbrink and Mr. Ho Ky Minh, Da Nang People's Committee vice chairman, provided formal remarks during the ceremony, which was accompanied by military courtesies and protocol standard for such events.

Due to the dangerous sea state and the resulting inability to get members of the media safely to TR immediately after the press conference, approximately 65 reporters visited BKH for one hour to film b-roll footage and capture still imagery the next day. Reporters toured the bridge, hangar bay, fo'c'sle, aft missile deck, and other areas of the ship. Outlets in attendance included Reuters, Channel News Asia, Dat Viet Newspaper, Tuoi Tre Newspaper, VN Express, and Da Nang Newspaper.

On Saturday, March 7th, a group of 30 reporters traveled by boat to TR for a tour of the hangar bay and flight deck. This was the only group to visit TR for a tour of the ship during the port visit. Due to the dangerous sea state and the resulting inability for other tour groups to visit TR safely, ship tours were shifted to BKH. 400 guests from the local Border Guard, Vietnam People's Navy, Military Region, municipal government, Vietnam Veterans, and American Chamber of Commerce visited the cruiser between March 5th and March 6th.[114]

COVID-19 concerns impacted other planned port visit events as well. The Government of Vietnam cancelled shipboard tours for 100 additional guests on Sunday, March 8th. The U.S. Pacific Fleet band modified their performance schedule in accordance with Vietnamese direction to refrain from large public gatherings. However, the band performed at several events, including a Vietnamese-hosted dinner, a Charity Center COMREL, a CPF-hosted reception, a Hoa Mai Orphanage COMREL and an event at the Nguyen Huu Dinh Opera Theatre.

---

[114] TR AAR For 5-9 March Vietnam PVST dtd 17 Mar 20

Three planned professional exchanges, in which Vietnamese air traffic controllers, firefighting personnel and meteorologists would have toured TR were cancelled due to sea state and/or COVID-19 concerns. U.S. Country Team representatives supported a Humanitarian Assistance and Disaster Relief (HA/DR) professional exchange ashore, focusing on disease prevention at Da Nang Hospital for Women and Children. Members of the media attended, but CSG-9 members did not.

During the port visit, concerns regarding COVID-19 rose at all levels. On March 4th, both Thailand and Vietnam were classified as HPCON "A" (Normal) with a Department of State Advisory Level "1" (practice usual precautions). On March 6th, Exercise COBRA GOLD (a joint combined Navy/Army/USMC event) concluded in Thailand, involving 4,500 U.S. personnel.[115] None of those personnel developed COVID-19.[116]

On March 8th, the Vietnamese Government notified CSG-9 that Sailors may have been exposed to COVID-19 during a stay at the Vanda Hotel in Da Nang, because two British citizens who had been guests of that hotel had tested positive for COVID-19.[117] TR and BKH suspended liberty for the remainder of the day, and ultimately the remainder of the port visit.[118] All remaining planned tours and professional engagements were cancelled. TR's Public Affairs Officer (PAO) (Command Duty Officer on March 8th) set up an emergency command center in the Strike Operations center aboard TR and information was gathered to form a list of people who stayed or had interactions at the Vanda Hotel grounds.[119] TR leadership quickly identified the location of 37 Sailors known to have stayed at the hotel. Of those, 11 TR Sailors identified as having stayed at and still present at the hotel were screened, tested on-site, and released to TR for quarantine. 26 other TR Sailors identified as having stayed at the hotel, but no longer there were removed from TR to the pier, screened, tested and returned to TR for quarantine. Later that day, two additional Sailors reported to TR medical staff that they had also visited the hotel. These two Sailors were not tested, but were quarantined on TR. All 39 Sailors remained in quarantine[120] for 14 days. TR remained at anchor one additional day due to sea state, and on March 9th, departed Da Nang.

---

[115] The 39th Iteration of Cobra Gold Concludes with a Combined Arms-Live Fire Exercise and Closing Ceremony *U.S. Army Public Affairs Office* (6 Mar 20) https://www.army.mil/article/233549/cobra_gold_20_the_39th_iteration_of_cobra_gold_concludes_with_a_combined_arms_live_fire _exercise_and_closing_ceremony
[116] C7F COS Statement dtd 21 May 20; Email – C7F – Response to RFI dtd 15 May 20
[117] Crozier, B. CAPT Statement dtd 15 May 20
[118] Crozier, B. CAPT Statement dtd 15 May 20
[119] TR CDO Report dtd 8 Mar 20
[120] Crozier, B. CAPT Statement dtd 15 May 20

## Chapter 3 – Actions during USS Theodore Roosevelt Transit to and Arrival in Guam

Underway Quarantine and Initial COVID-19 Positive Sailors Aboard TR

On March 9[th], TR got underway from anchorage in Da Nang Bay, Vietnam, with 39 Sailors in quarantine (see Figures 2 and 3), and resumed normal operations in the C7F area of operations. At this time, with the exception of the quarantined area, the entire operational chain of command believed that TR was a COVID-free ship.

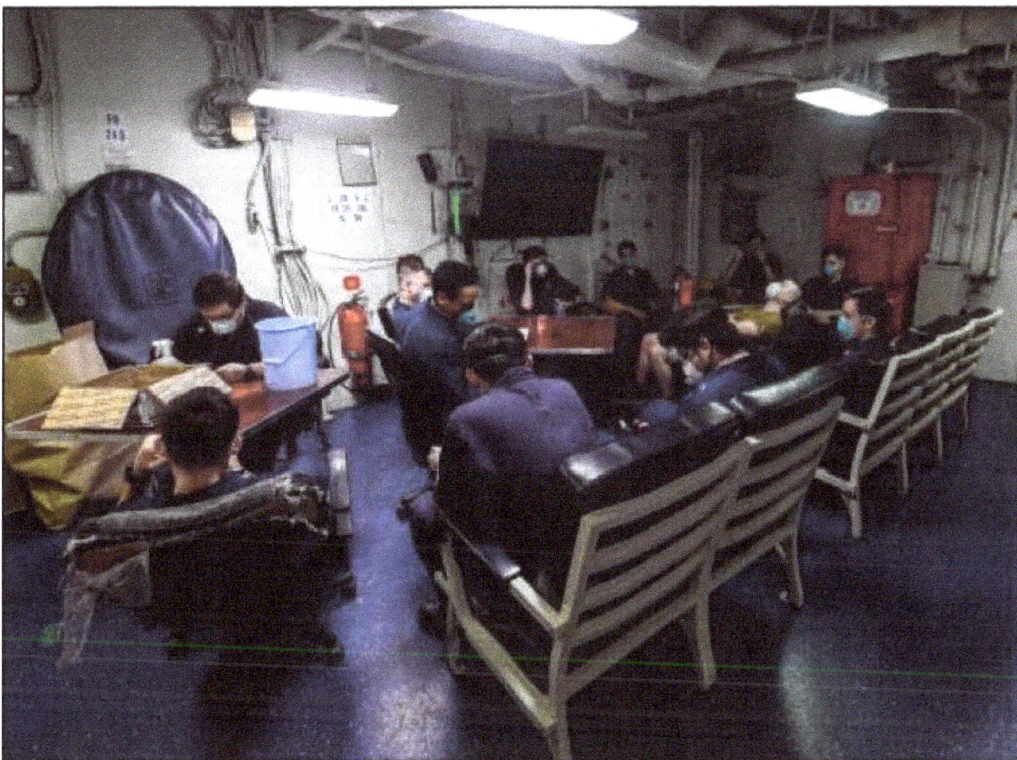

*Figure 2: 200521-N-SH180-3010 PHILIPPINE SEA (May 21, 2020) - U.S. Sailors sit in a crew lounge area that was one of the first quarantine spaces aboard USS Theodore Roosevelt (CVN 71). (U.S. Navy photo by Mass Communication Specialist 3rd Class Zachary Wheeler)*

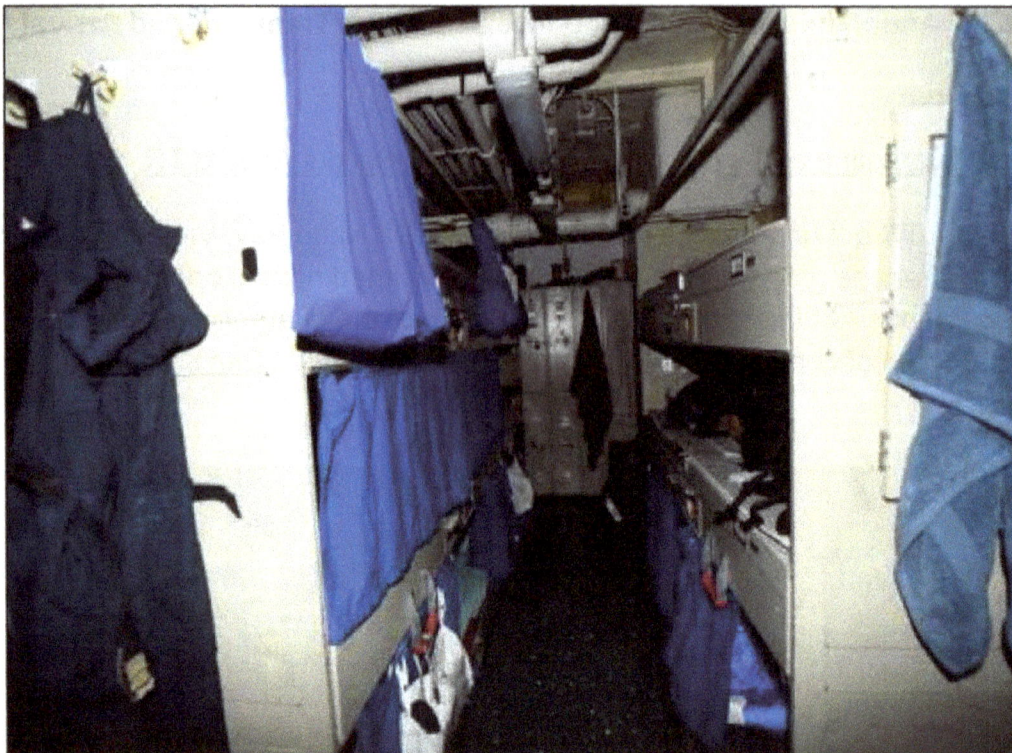

*Figure 3. 2200521-N-SH180-3014 PHILIPINE SEA (May 21, 2020) – A reactor berthing compartment that was one of the first quarantine spaces aboard USS Theodore Roosevelt (CVN 71).*
*(U.S. Navy photo by Mass Communication Specialist 3rd Class Zachary Wheeler)*

The outbreak of norovirus earlier in the deployment resulted in a continuing effort to clean common touch areas throughout the ship with an appropriate disinfecting agent. The crew used bleach solution, approved for shipboard use, to clean the ship daily. All ship's services continued as usual. The ship's crew received daily reminders to wash their hands, maintain social distancing, and not touch their faces. These messages were delivered in several ways: TR's XO made daily announcements on the public address system (1MC) and the TR CO made similar announcements every other day. Department Heads received information to inform their department personnel, and the medical staff created a video that was broadcast continuously on the ship's closed-circuit television channel. Additionally, in compliance with guidance at the time, the TR SMO had every department conduct verbal COVID-19 screenings of all Sailors (asking for flu-like symptoms: fever, chills, cough, sore throat, shortness of breath and body aches) daily for a period of seven days. After March 16th, Sailors were requested to self-assess and report to Medical if having any symptoms.[121]

TR's CO restricted self-service on the main galley lines on March 9th, however self-service remained an option for other food selections such as the salad bar.

---

[121] Email - TR SMO to All Officers, All CPOs, All E-6 and below - 14 days of screening following port visits dtd 16 Mar 20

During the transit, the TR communicated to the medical and operational chains of command that they were unable to fully comply with the requirements contained in the C7F TASKORD (C7F TASKORD for Force Health Protection against COVID-19).[122] CPF and C7F Fleet Surgeons requested TR continue to do the screening they were conducting.[123]

From the time the ship left Da Nang on March 9th until March 23rd, seven COD flights originating out of Clark Air Force Base in the Philippines brought a total of 29 passengers and COD detachment personnel to the carrier.[124] All 29 screened negative for COVID-19 symptoms upon their arrival,[125] following the screening protocols required by the February 23, 2020 C7F FRAGORD.[126] Later, four of those personnel tested positive for the virus, however the investigation team as well as the NMCPHC concluded that none of these Sailors were the likely source of the outbreak on TR (details in Appendix F).

From March 9th to March 23rd, up to nine Sailors presented to TR Medical with ILI symptoms. Sailors that presented with one or more ILI symptoms were screened by members of the embarked BDRD team for common respiratory pathogens using the BioFire Respiratory Panel (RP-2). If a positive test result was returned, the screening was halted. In each of these nine cases, a positive test result for common respiratory illnesses was returned.[127]

On March 23rd, TR stopped receiving COD flights from the Philippines.[128] The TR CO stated that due to the increasing number of COVID-19 cases in the Philippines, an internal decision was made to push all future passengers and parts to Kadena AFB or Anderson AFB and avoid further flights to the Philippines.[129] The investigation team concluded through analysis the following:

- Patients that presented with ILI symptoms prior to Da Nang were not likely COVID-19 positive cases.

- There is no indication that the virus came aboard TR via COD.

- There were indications of possibly undetected COVID cases aboard TR

[122] Email – TR SMO - Post-Danang Update dtd 17 Mar 20
[123] TR SMO Statement dtd 17 May 20; Email – TR SMO to CCSG-9 – Post-Danang update – dtd 18 Mar 20
[124] COD Completed Travel Log/Manifest
[125] Crozier, B. CAPT Statement dtd 15 May 20, TR XO Statement dtd 16 May 20; CVW-11 CAG Statement dtd 19 May 20
[126] TR SMO Statement dtd 17 May 20
[127] (b) (6) LCDR Statement dtd 23 May 20
[128] COD Completed Travel Log/Manifest
[129] Crozier, B. CAPT Statement dtd 15 May 20

following the Da Nang port visit.

A more detailed analysis of the probable source of COVID-19 on TR can be found in Appendix F of this report.

The prospective XO, who embarked prior to the ship's arrival in Da Nang, completed turnover with the outgoing TR XO, and officially assumed the role on March 11th.[130]

On March 13th, the TR CO sent letters to family members indicating the ship had begun COVID-19 testing for select individuals.[131] Members of Navy Forward-Deployed Preventive Medicine Units and Naval Medical Research Center, per the request of C7F, embarked TR[132] on March 14th while the 39 quarantined Sailors tested negative.[133] Members of the BDRD team tested the 39 Sailors on the Applied Biosystems Inc. StepOne Plus instrument, using the COVID-19 test, which had been approved for research-use only at that point.[134] Operations in 7th Fleet continued; USS Blue Ridge (LCC 19) arrived in Singapore for a previously scheduled port visit, Guam declared a state of public health emergency, even though no cases had yet been identified on Guam.[135]

On March 16th, the TR SMO emailed the crew of TR explaining that C7F released a revision to the Tasking Order (TASKORD) for Force Health Protection against COVID-19.[136] By March 17th, all 50 U.S. states had confirmed cases of the virus.[137] By March 20th, Guam had 12 confirmed cases of COVID.[138]

As TR prepared for their Guam port visit, scheduled for April 3rd – 10th, the TR CO and NBG CO correspondence regarding the same illustrated that TR was not seen as a COVID-threat to Guam, but significant efforts would need to be taken to ensure TR remained COVID-free, which would result in changes from their recent February port call to Guam.

On March 17th, the TR CO emailed[139] CO, NBG to propose three possible courses of action (COAs) for liberty during the TR's upcoming Guam port visit:

---

[130] Email - TR XO - TR Investigation dtd 8 May 20
[131] Crozier, B. CAPT Ltr to families dtd 13 Mar 20
[132] Navy Preventive Medicine Teams Embark Ships in 7th Fleet, *INDOPACOM*, (03 Mar 20) https://www.pacom.mil/Media/News/News-Article-View/Article/2122302/navy-preventive-medicine-teams-embark-ships-in-7th-fleet/
[133] Email - TR SMO - Post-Danang Update dtd 14 Mar 20
[134] (b) (6) LCDR Statement dtd 23 May 20
[135] Government of Guam Executive Order 2020-03
[136] Email - TR SMO - Coronavirus screening - Update dtd 16 Mar 20
[137] CORONAVIRUS: DOD RESPONSE TIMELINE (15 May 20) https://www.defense.gov/Explore/Spotlight/Coronavirus/DOD-Response-Timeline/
[138] Email - NBG CO to TR CO - TR PVST dtd 20 Mar 20
[139] Email - NBG CO to TR CO - TR PVST dtd 20 Mar 20

1. Full Guam liberty, similar to the previous port visit,

2. NBG liberty with base access (busses to Navy Exchange (NEX), beach, etc.), and limited off-base liberty (golf, small group tours, etc.),

3. Or pier liberty with limited access to NBG (busses to NEX, beach, etc.) and MWR pier support (food/beer/entertainment/wifi).

CO, NBG responded that Guam now had 12 confirmed COVID-19 cases and although none of the cases were on base, he deemed that the possibility of exposure on base to the TR was a threat for their port visit and forwarded NAVBASE Guam Notice 6210, "U.S. Naval Base Guam Maritime Vessel Quarantine Procedures for a Clean Ship." CO, NBG stated that only COA 3 was appropriate and that further mitigation measures were needed to afford TR Sailors access to the NEX and that TR medical personnel would be required to assist in screening and sanitization inspections.[140]

On March 22nd, TR CO emailed CO, NBG and provided a summary of the TR liberty plan for the upcoming Guam port visit that complied with the limitations of COA 3. TR CO outlined in detail that liberty would be confined to the pier with limited NBG access. He requested support equipment and supplies for beer sales, barbeques, Wi-Fi, and games. In addition to pier activities, TR CO requested exclusive access to Gab Gab beach for TR Sailors with the availability of MWR rental equipment such as paddleboards and volleyball. TR CO requested limited access to NBG locations such as the NEX, Liberty Center, movie theater, gym, ballfields, and hiking areas.[141]

CO, NBG responded to TR CO that his first priority was the safe mooring of the ship and proper husbanding while in port, all while ensuring that the ship and crew remained "clean." He stated that "once we have that locked in we will focus on the quality of life." CO, NBG attached the below general schematic for Kilo Wharf (Figure 4) and the potential Force Health Protection Enclave (FHPE) that would be employed to enable the required separation for TR Sailors to base support personnel.[142]

[140] Email - NBG CO to TR CO - TR PVST dtd 20 Mar 20
[141] Email – NBG CO to TR CO - RE TR PVST dtd 23 Mar 20
[142] Email – NBG CO to TR CO - RE TR PVST dtd 23 Mar 20

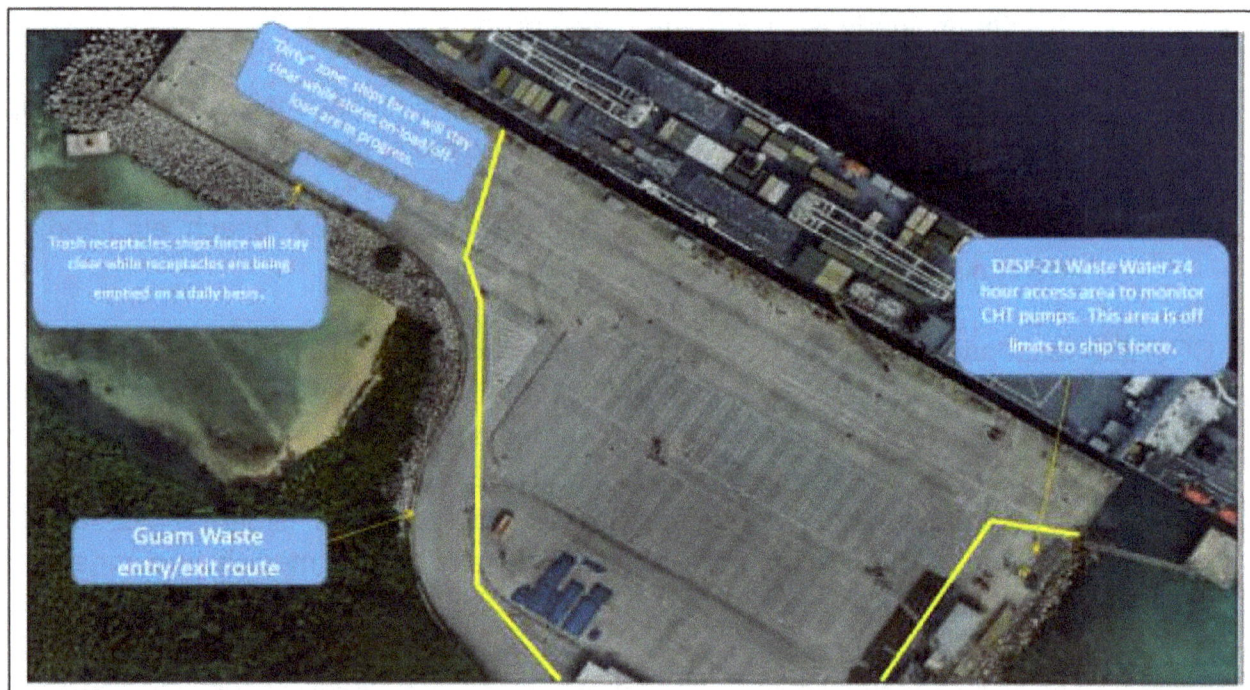

Figure 4. Kilo Wharf, Naval Base Guam, laydown for TR's arrival on March 27, 2020.

## First COVID-Positive Tests

On March 22nd, after a 14-day quarantine period, all 39 Sailors potentially exposed to COVID-19 in Da Nang remained asymptomatic, tested negative for COVID-19 a third time, and were released from quarantine.[143]  However, on March 23rd, two Sailors, both from the air wing, began showing COVID-19 symptoms.[144]  Those two, and an additional Sailor from the nuclear reactor department, tested positive for COVID-19 on March 24th.[145]  None of these three Sailors were among the 39 who had been potentially exposed to the virus in Da Nang and subsequently placed in quarantine.

From this point forward, despite no known COVID cases aboard, the ship did not implement actions such as enforcing social distancing measures on the mess decks[146] (i.e., no seats were removed, lines continued to form without six feet of separation between Sailors and condiments were available for common use).[147]  Gyms, chapel, and ship's store remained open.

---

[143] C7F COS Statement dtd 21 May 20; Crozier, B. CAPT Statement dtd 15 May 20; TR XO Statement dtd 16 May 20; TR SMO Statement dtd 17 May 20; C7F Surgeon Statement dtd 23 May 20

[144] Email (SIPR) - CCSG-9 to C7F and C3F - POSITIVE COVID-19 TESTS ON TR (initial report) dtd 24 Mar 20

[145] Email (SIPR) - CCSG-9 - Positive COVID-19 tests on TR (update #9) dtd 26 Mar 20; Email - TR SMO to CCSG-9 - COVID 19 update 24 March dtd 24 Mar 20, 0440

[146] AME1 Statement dtd 13 May 20; CSC Statement dtd.13 May 20; TR CMC Statement dtd 17 May 20

[147] Email - TR SMO to TR CO – Follow Up dtd 9 Mar 20; TR SUPPO Statement dtd 18 May 20; TR XO Statement dtd 16 May 20

## Planning for Arrival in Guam

As TR confirmed the first Sailors with COVID-19 aboard TR, two commercial cruise ships, Diamond Princess and Grand Princess, were experiencing more than 800 total COVID-19 cases while at sea, including 10 deaths. As the first U.S. Navy warship to have a COVID outbreak underway, CSG-9 and TR leadership paid close attention to observations from the cruise ship Diamond Princess and other cruise ships experiencing COVID outbreaks. They recognized two significant differences between Diamond Princess and TR. First, berthing onboard TR was primarily open bay group berthing with shared heads, while the Diamond Princess berthing was comprised mainly of staterooms (accommodating one or two people). Secondly, the demographics of the ships were different. TR had a younger, healthier population, while Diamond Princess had an older demographic. Cruise ships were experiencing difficulty in obtaining authorization from host nations to enter port and in the case of the Diamond Princess and Grand Princess, required extraordinary levels of support to manage the movement of embarked guests ashore. Guam had denied entry to cruise ship MS WESTERDAM over COVID-19 concerns on February 7th, even though there were no known COVID-positive people aboard.[148]

TR was originally scheduled for a port visit to Guam from April 3rd to April 10th.[149] On March 25th, TR sailed for Guam at USS Bunker Hill's best speed based on maximum allowable fuel burn rate for the planned transit[150] and TR sent a logistics request (LOGREQ) for a March 27th arrival in Guam.

C7F suggested using the ship's hangar deck for segregated berthing, and considered flying the Command Element and the air wing off the ship to Anderson Air Force Base, Guam. Anderson Air Force Base had significant concerns about COVID-positive patients flying to that base.[151] Commander, Task Force (CTF) 75 offered tents with air conditioning and cots for 400 Sailors to be available on the pier if needed.[152] After the third Sailor tested positive for COVID-19, the TR CO conducted a 1MC call informing the crew that antiseptic wipes and hand sanitizer were available throughout the ship, that self-service was secured on the mess decks, the Chief Petty Officers' mess and wardrooms, dental services were now limited, and "bleach-a-palooza" would occur twice daily.[153] C7F was aware of the preventive measures currently being taken aboard

[148] Guam denies entry to ship over coronavirus concerns, *USA Today* (07 Feb 20) https://www.usatoday.com/story/news/local/2020/02/07/guam-denies-entry-ship-over-coronavirus-concerns/4687803002/
[149] Email - CSG-9 – Response to RFI dtd 20 May 20
[150] Crozier, B. CAPT Statement dtd 15 May 20; C7F COS Statement dtd 16 May 20; , TR XO Statement dtd 16 May 20; TR RO Statement dtd 18 May 20
[151] Email (SIPR) – C7F to CCSG-9, C7F CoS, CSG-9 CoS – RE: (S) Positive COVID tests on TR (Update #2) dtd 24 Mar 20
[152] Email (SIPR) – CTF 75 to C7F – COVID-19 Commander's perspective 22 Mar dtd 24 Mar 20
[153] Email – TR PAO – TRSG RTQ dtd 24 Mar 20 0149 (containing 200323 TRSG Positive COVID 1MC Remarks)

TR.[154] The SMO requested assistance from Navy Medicine upon arrival in Guam.[155] C7F and CPF Fleet Surgeons concurred with the SMO that at this point "anyone who is defined as [having influenza-like illness symptoms] is a presumptive [positive] COVID-19 and should be treated as such."[156]

By March 25th, TR had four Sailors positive for COVID-19, and moved them ashore to Naval Hospital Guam via helicopter.[157] On March 25th, the CSG-9 COS notified the C7F COS of the need for 4,000 rooms to house Sailors in single isolation for two weeks.[158]

As COVID-19 cases rose to eight,[159] the TR CO sent letters to family members indicating "a few Sailors" had tested positive for COVID-19, had been placed in isolation, and work was in progress to fly those Sailors off the ship as soon as possible.[160] (Figures 5 and 6 depict Sailors working aboard the ship using social distancing measures).

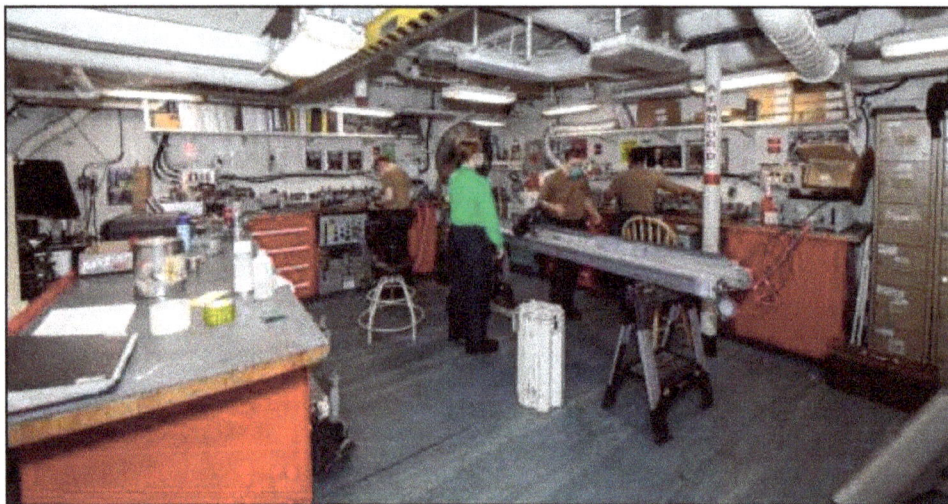

*Figure 5: 200521-N-MQ442-1006 PHILIPPINE SEA (May 21, 2020) -- U.S. Sailors work in the aviation ordnance shop aboard the aircraft carrier USS Theodore Roosevelt (CVN 71). Seven Sailors typically work in this space. (U.S. Navy photo by Mass Communication Specialist 3rd Class Dartañon D. De La Garza)*

---

[154] Email – C7F PAO to TR PAO – FWD: Proposed Statement dtd 26 Mar 20
[155] Email – TR SMO to CPF and C7F Fleet Surgeons - WARNORD for BUMED dtd 24 Mar 20
[156] Email – TR SMO to CPF and C7F Fleet Surgeons - WARNORD for BUMED dtd 24 Mar 20
[157] CO NHG Statement dtd 18 May 20; Sailors tested positive on USS Theodore Roosevelt, extent of exposure unclear, *Pacific Daily News* (23 Mar 20) https://www.guampdn.com/story/news/local/2020/03/26/sailors-tested-positive-uss-roosevelt-extent-exposure-unclear/5084652002/#
[158] Email (SIPR) – CSG-9 COS to C7F COS – HOTEL OPTION dtd 25 Mar 20
[159] Eight sailors from USS Theodore Roosevelt have coronavirus, raising concerns about pandemic's strain on military, *USA Today* (24 Mar 20) https://www.usatoday.com/story/news/politics/2020/03/24/coronavirus-3-sailors-test-positive-military-readiness-affected/2910165001
[160] Email – Crozier, B. CAPT to TR Ombudsmen – TR letter to families – with Letter to TR Families and Friends dtd 24 Mar 20

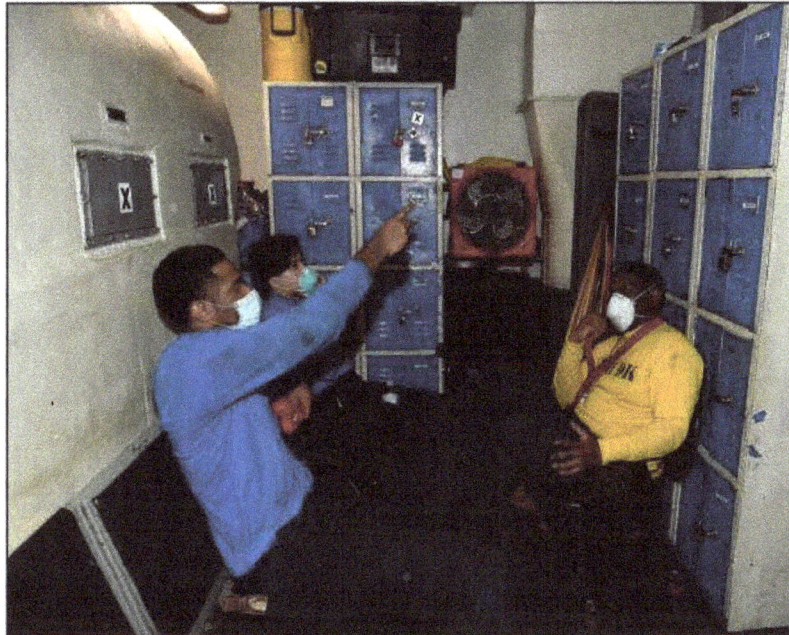

*Figure 6: 200521-N-XX200-2116 PHILIPPINE SEA (MAY 21, 2020) - U.S. Sailors work in an Air Department work center aboard the aircraft carrier USS Theodore Roosevelt (CVN 71). Up to eight Sailors typically work in this space. (US Navy photo by Mass Communication Specialist Seaman Erik Melgar)*

TR's positive COVID-19 cases grew from eight to 33 by March 26th.[161] With numbers of cases increasing, C7F continued coordinating efforts to develop a plan for disembarking TR Sailors. During a discussion with C7F, the Commanding General of III Marine Expeditionary Force (III MEF) offered up to 5,000 rooms for potential occupancy in Okinawa.[162] An email from CO, NBG to the C7F COS and CSG-9 COS detailed a plan for TR's arrival to Guam and provided the slides in figures 7 through 9 below.[163] The priority after safely mooring was to transport Sailors who were COVID-19 positive and 20 Reactor Department Sailors (key watchstanders who were being protected as backups and kept in reserve) to isolation rooms. CO, NBG's scheme of maneuver brief shows the availability of 150 isolation beds and 493 quarantine beds in gyms and open bay facilities upon TR's expected March 27th arrival.[164]

---

[161] Email (SIPR) – CCSG-9 - Positive COVID-19 tests on TR (update #9) dtd 26 Mar 20
[162] C7F Statement dtd 18 May 20
[163] Email (SIPR) – CO NBG – NBG Task Force TR REVIVE dtd 26 Mar 20
[164] Email (SIPR) – CO NBG – NBG Task Force TR REVIVE dtd 26 Mar 20

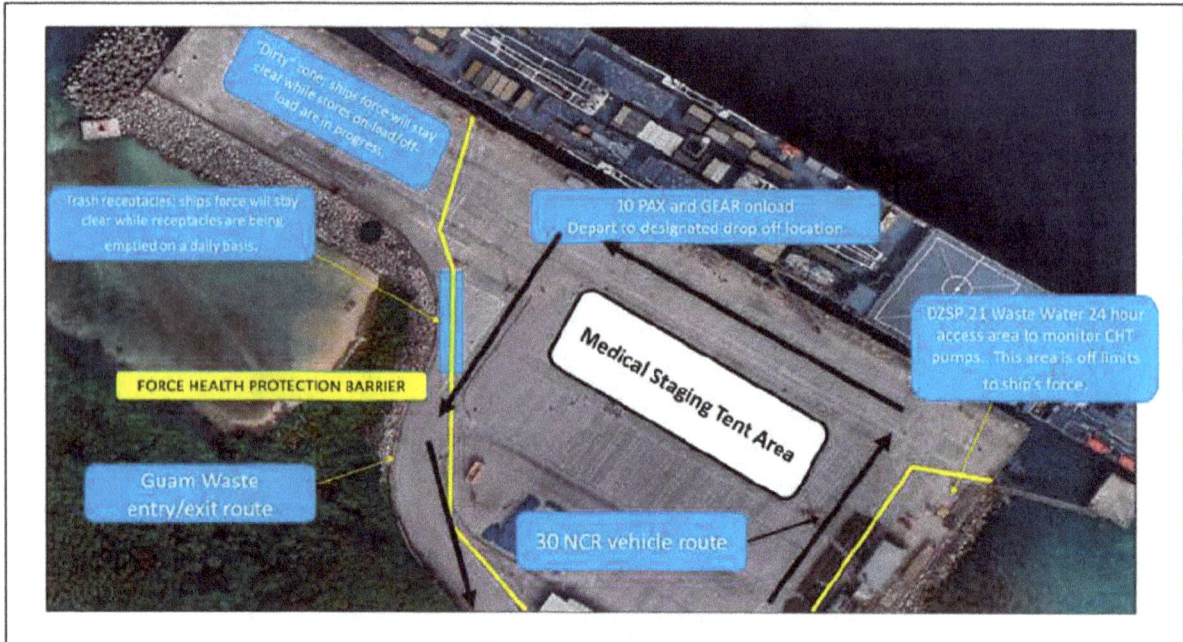

Figure 7:  Kilo Wharf Laydown[165]

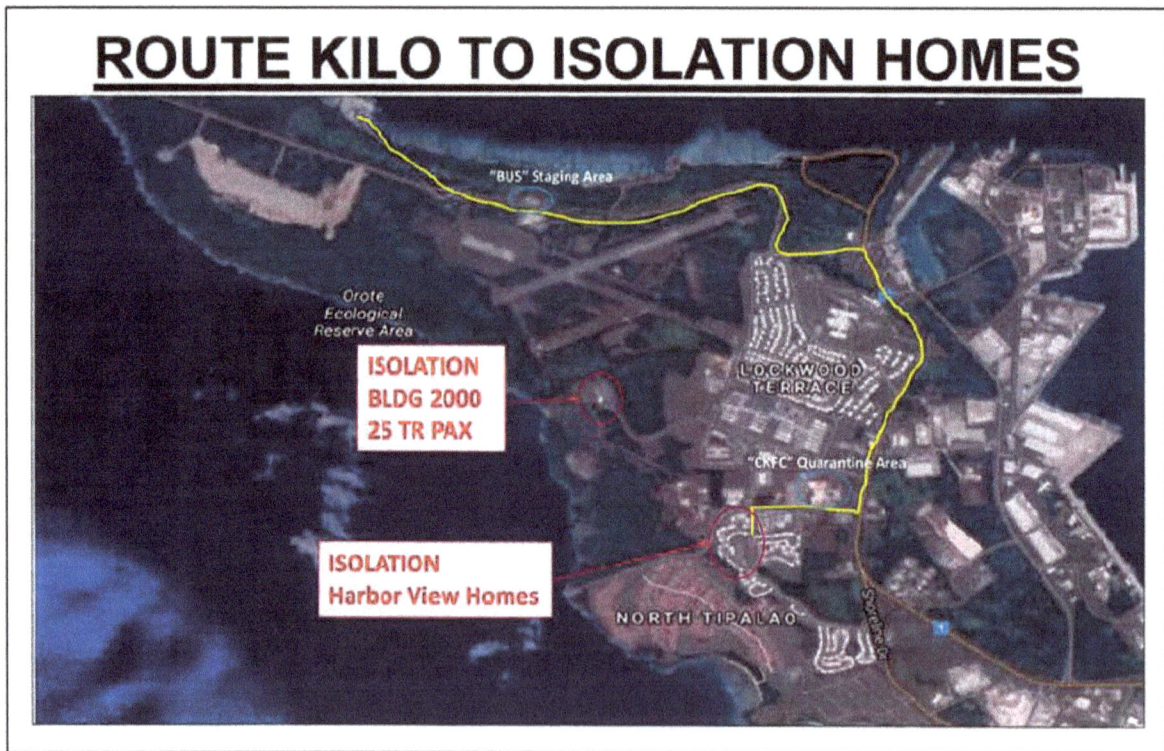

Figure 8:  Route to Isolation Homes[166]

[165] Email (SIPR) – CO NBG – NBG Task Force TR REVIVE dtd 26 Mar 20
[166] Email (SIPR) – CO NBG – NBG Task Force TR REVIVE dtd 26 Mar 20

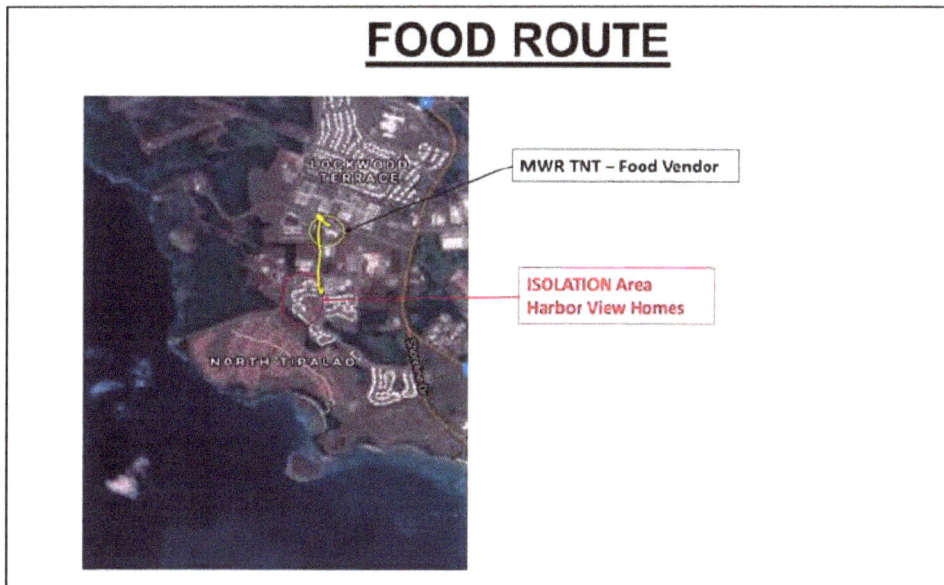

Figure 9: Food Route[167]

Navy published definitions of quarantine and isolation, derived from CDC guidance, on March 23rd.[168] Quarantine referred to the separation of a person or group from others as a result of suspected exposure to a communicable disease to prevent its spread. Quarantine was to be imposed on those with no COVID-19 symptoms who had either recently returned from a high-risk location (CDC Travel Health Notice Level 2 or 3), or had close contact with a known COVID-19 positive person. The recommended quarantine period was 14 days. The same Navy guidance defined isolation as the separation of a person or group from others due either to the development of potential COVID-19 symptoms or as a result of a positive COVID-19 test. A third definition of Restrictions on Movement (ROM) applied to personnel directed to remain at home or in a comparable setting for 14 days from the day of contact with a COVID-19 positive person. For transient personnel and those residing in close quarters such as unaccompanied housing or ships, temporary lodging meeting CDC guidance of separate sleeping and bathroom facilities shall be arranged, when available.

On March 26th, CCSG-9 issued Commander's Guidance to the strike group for arrival in Guam expressing the following priorities:

1. move all COVID-positive Sailors to isolation quarters;

2. identify key groups needed to operate ship at sea in near-term;

---

[167] Email (SIPR) – CO NBG – NBG Task Force TR REVIVE dtd 26 Mar 20
[168] NAVADMIN 083/20 Restriction of Movement (ROM) Guidance 23 Mar 20

3. move key reactor supervisory personnel into isolation following testing; and

4. if additional quarantine racks remain, prioritize by personnel and by function.

The desired near-term end state was to have sufficient personnel to get the ship underway for contingency operations.[169] This was a reasonable and appropriate set of priorities given the size of the outbreak at the time and the limited knowledge of what COVID-19 PCR testing could actually do.

As concern for TR elevated up operational and administrative chains of command, CPF emailed the first of a series of TR Recovery and Disposition Plan updates to the four-star admiral commanding U.S. Indo-Pacific Command (INDOPACOM) and to the CNO. CPF noted that the plan was to test the entire TR crew for COVID-19.[170]

On March 26th, C7F emailed the Deputy Chief of Naval Operations (DCNO) for Operations, Plans and Strategy (N3/N5) recommending Echelon I engagement and support for additional resources for testing 100 percent of the TR crew.[171] The C7F COS stated that testing before moving to quarantine was not required and that C7F was clear to CCSG-9 that the intent was to move Sailors ashore as fast as possible.[172]

With one day remaining before TR's arrival in Guam, CCSG-9 emailed C7F that TR would run out of quarantine and isolation space ashore in Guam. Adding complexity to the situation, an email response from the CNO to CPF stated his understanding that 100 percent of the crew would be tested and a response on the same email thread from C7F stated that "100 percent was desired but likely not possible." In the same email thread, the DCNO (OPNAV N3/N5), who was responsible for Navy's overall plan to combat COVID-19, replied to C7F that the "Crew of TR will not leave pier, with the exception of positive Sailors, who will be sequestered in base berthing facilities." The email thread continued the same day with the CNO again stating for clarification to CPF that he understood that CPF's intent was 100 percent testing for the TR crew.[173] On March 28th, C7F emailed CCSG-9 to address an earlier conversation in which CCSG-9 reported he was sending Sailors to ashore quarantine without an initial test. C7F stated in his email, "You get no credit for those folks."[174] CCSG-9 replied, "Copy all and WILCO," implying he now understood a 100 percent testing requirement for Sailors to move ashore.[175] This perceived direction from higher authority was in opposition to the

---

[169] Email (SIPR) – CCSG-9 to Crozier, B. CAPT, CVW-11 CAG – (S) OUTBREAK COMMANDER'S GUIDANCE dtd 26 Mar 20
[170] Email (SIPR) – CPF to CNO and INDOPACOM - TR Recovery and Disposition Plan dtd 26 Mar 20
[171] Email (SIPR) – C7F to OPNAV N3/N5 – RE: (U//FOUO) FOR INFORMATION: TR Recovery and Disposition Plan dtd 26 Mar 20
[172] C7F COS Statement dtd 16 May 20
[173] Email (SIPR) – N3/5 to C7F – RE: (U//FOUO) FOR INFORMATION: TR Recovery and Disposition Plan dtd 26 Mar 20
[174] Email (SIPR) - C7F to CCSG-9 – SUBJ: (S) 28 Mar TB - follow-up dtd 28 Mar 20
[175] Email (SIPR) - C7F to CCSG-9 – SUBJ: (S) 28 Mar TB - follow-up dtd 28 Mar 20

plan to remove the healthy 840 "Tier I" personnel needed to steam the ship and caused further confusion among the warfare commanders.[176]

Arrival and Initial Disembarkation

On March 27th, TR arrived in Guam and moored at the pier[177] with 36 COVID-19 positive Sailors aboard the carrier.  Upon arrival, CCSG-9 and TR planned to rapidly move both confirmed COVID-positive Sailors and key watchstanders known to have avoided contact with any positive Sailors off the ship.  264 Sailors moved ashore to available berthing according to this plan.  There was no plan at this time to move ashore the large number of Sailors quarantined on the ship, nor was there clarity on testing requirements prior to sending Sailors ashore to NBG.  Compounding the confusion, the C7F COS emphasized to CSG-9 that all people must be tested before they leave the ship.[178]

TR closed the remaining gyms aboard ship once in port and created a pier gym for Sailor use.[179]  Creation of this pier gym was inconsistent with published Navy and Fleet guidance.  Additionally, the ship continued to conduct Command Urinalysis screening despite the release of Navy guidance[180] on March 27th (NAVADMIN date – March 28th Guam) authorizing commanding officers to pause the program in response to the strict enforcement of social distancing measures.[181]  In contrast, Navy facilities ashore and units at sea had by this date (March 24th) secured gyms and religious services and mandated social distancing in dining facilities consistent with NAVADMIN 080/20 released on March 22nd.[182]

As the TR arrived in Guam, C7F said he was "crystal clear" to CCSG-9 that C7F wanted as many Sailors off the ship as quickly as possible.[183]  Once CPF received word that Korea could test 1,000 samples per day, CPF directed testing of TR's entire crew.[184]  In order to do this, CPF directed getting the entire crew tested, the ship cleaned and declared clear of the virus as soon as possible so the crew could get back to the ship and get underway.[185]  The fastest means to achieve this was to establish a testing rate

---

[176] CVW-11 CAG Statement dtd 19 May 20; Crozier, B. CAPT Statement dtd 15 May 20; Email – CVW-11 CAG to CCSG-9 – PROPOSED PAPER / COURSE OF ACTION FROM WARFARE COMMANDERS dtd 29 Mar 20
[177] Facebook Post - Family and Friends of the Rough Riders, Crozier, B. CAPT (27 Mar 20)
https://www.facebook.com/USSTheodoreRoosevelt/photos/a.489137065779/10156700551025780/?type=3&theater
[178] Email (SIPR) - C7F COS to COS CSG-9 - Triage and Procedure dtd 27 Mar 20
[179] Email – TR Afloat Rec Specialist – Gym's Secured dtd 29 Mar 20
[180] NAVADMIN 092/20 Urinalysis Policy Update dtd 27 Mar 20
[181] TR MA2 to TR Crew - URINALYSIS POLICY UPDATE dtd 29 Mar 20
[182] NAVADMIN 080/20 Navy Mitigation Measures in Response to Coronavirus Outbreak Update 3 dtd 21 Mar 20
[183] C7F COS Statement dtd 16 May 20
[184] C7F COS Statement dtd 16 May 20
[185] C7F COS Interview dtd 16 May 20

of 500 tests per day to match available shipboard testing capacity, as a goal. Upon arrival, TR could only swab approximately 200 Sailors per day without outside medical support personnel.[186] C7F stated that they were aware of the testing capacity limitation as well as ongoing efforts to supply sufficient swabs, however they felt continual pressure from CPF to attain the 500 per day goal, and to ultimately expand to the advertised capacity of 1,000 per day for the lab in Korea.[187] CCSG-9 and TR felt continuous pressure from these requirements, and they felt distracted from egressing the crew in a timely manner. There was no meaningful discussion at leadership meetings on when these samples should be taken – before leaving the ship or after. TR was executing the samples before allowing Sailors to leave. C7F said he believed TR was "slow-rolling" Sailors leaving the ship. In contrast, TR and CCSG-9 leaders viewed the testing as an unnecessary distraction.[188]

While CCSG-9's guidance established movement of COVID-19 infected Sailors to isolation ashore as the first priority, the next priority was preserving the ability to get underway rapidly for contingency operations, and accordingly key watchstanders that had been protected from spread of infection were quarantined next. The lack of clarity about available facilities ashore and plans for testing Sailors aboard ship contributed to delays in getting potentially non-infected crewmembers off the ship.[189]

On March 28th, TR's CO sent letters to family members announcing the ship's arrival in Guam. He indicated that Sailors with positive test results or symptoms indicative of COVID-19 were the first priority to get off the ship for evaluation at NBG Hospital. He further stated that some Sailors would be moved to open bay berthing off the ship and that parts of the ship would be used to quarantine "close contact" Sailors.[190]

The same day, TR received new higher capacity COVID-19 testing kits, but they required 12-14 days of preparation before use.[191] After previously stressing that all Sailors would be tested prior to departing the ship, CCSG-9 decided to move people off the ship as quickly as possible and test later.[192] The ship worked to batch-test 200 people who had already moved ashore before the ship was able to test them. A batch test ran the samples of multiple Sailors at once enabling the medical team to determine if a COVID-19 case was in the tested group. A batch test does not individually diagnose Sailors. If a batch were to test positive for COVID-19, the medical team would take

[186] Email – TR SMO to CSG-9 Staff – Testing Planning Factors dtd 27 Mar 20
[187] Email – C7F COS– RE: Signed C7F COS statement dtd 22 May 20
[188] Email – CVW-11 CAG to CCSG-9 – PROPOSED PAPER / COURSE OF ACTION FROM WARFARE COMMANDERS dtd 29 Mar 20
[189] Crozier, B. CAPT Statement dtd 15 May 20; TR XO Statement dtd 16 May 20
[190] Email – Crozier, B. CAPT to TR Ombudsmen – (none) with Letter to TR Families and Friends dtd 24 Mar 20
[191] Email (SIPR) – CNO to CPF – INFO TR recovery and disposition update 27 Mar 20 dtd 28 Mar 20
[192] Email (SIPR) – CCSG-9 - 28 Mar TB - follow up dtd 28 Mar 20

additional measures, such as isolating the Sailors whose samples were in the batch, and depending on the Sailor's symptoms, potentially medically evacuating them off the ship to a shore facility for testing.[193]

Providing food for the number of TR Sailors ashore in isolation and quarantine was a challenge.[194] As the number of Sailors ashore increased, the contracted food delivery had difficulty keeping up with the increasing demand. TR Sailors complained of problems[195] that leadership addressed as quickly as they could. Sailors expressed their concerns on social media and this was relayed to the TR CO and TR XO.[196] Contributing to this sense of "helplessness," NBG did not allow (at the time) any TR supervisors to review the temporary facilities for their Sailors, but neither did TR leadership address this with NBG or others.[197]

The ship's leaders were also concerned that the temporary open-bay facilities did not meet CDC guidelines and cots were not initially arranged to enable social distancing. In reaction to the social media posts and out of concern about the living conditions ashore, the TR CO established policy that no Sailors would leave the ship until guarantee of sufficient meal service was available.[198] Additionally, the CO requested the ability for ship's company to inspect isolation and quarantine facilities for suitability prior to moving Sailors (e.g., adequate meal service, heads, and physical separation).[199] Figures 10 through 14 below depict a sampling of the shore facilities in place for TR Sailors.

---

[193] Navy Preventive Medicine Teams Embark Ships in 7th Fleet, *INDOPACOM*, (03 Mar 20) https://www.pacom.mil/Media/News/News-Article-View/Article/2122302/navy-preventive-medicine-teams-embark-ships-in-7th-fleet/
[194] NBG CO statement dtd 18 May 20; TR XO Statement dtd 16 May 20
[195] AME2 Statement dtd 16 May 20; AN Statement dtd 16 May 20; TR CMC Statement dtd 17 May 20; TR XO Statement dtd 16 May 20
[196] Crozier, B. CAPT Statement dtd 15 May 20; TR XO Statement dtd 16 May 20; TR PAO Interview Summary dtd 23 May 20
[197] Crozier, B. CAPT Statement dtd 15 May 20
[198] Crozier, B. CAPT Statement dtd 15 May 20; TR XO Statement dtd 16 May 20
[199] Crozier, B. CAPT Statement dtd 15 May 20; TR CMC Statement dtd 17 May 20

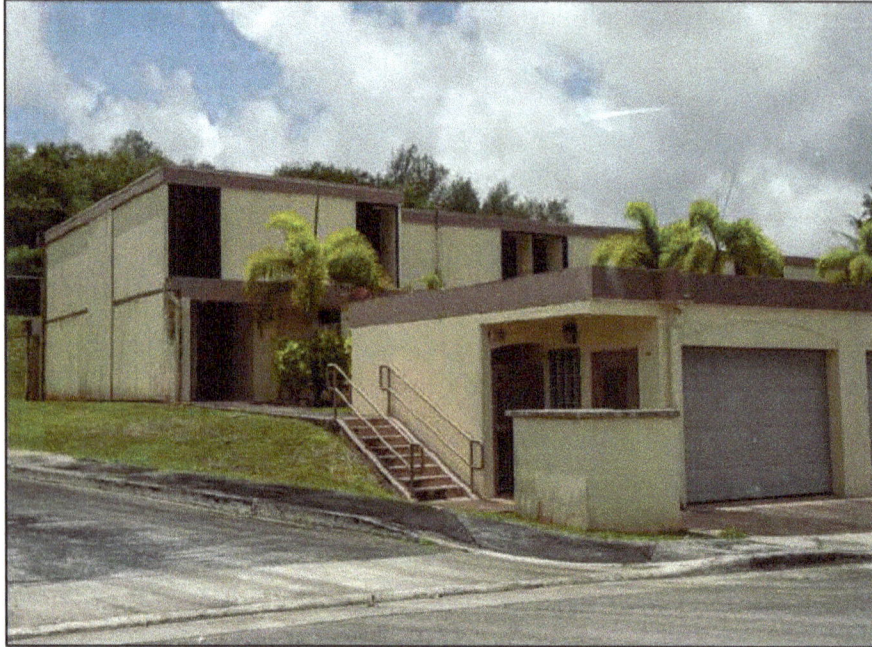

Figure 10: Vacant Family Housing in Guam

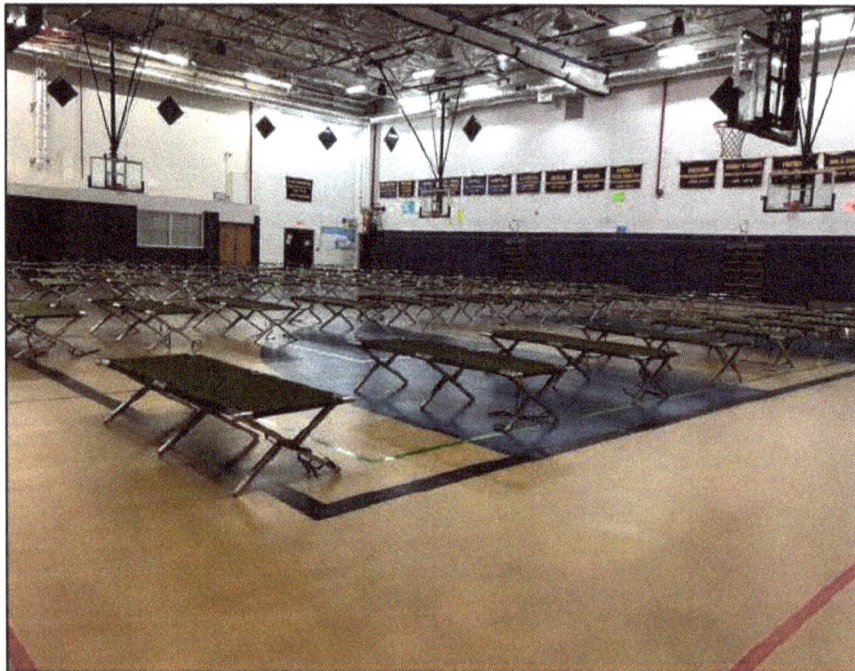

Figure 11: Gym Cot Setup

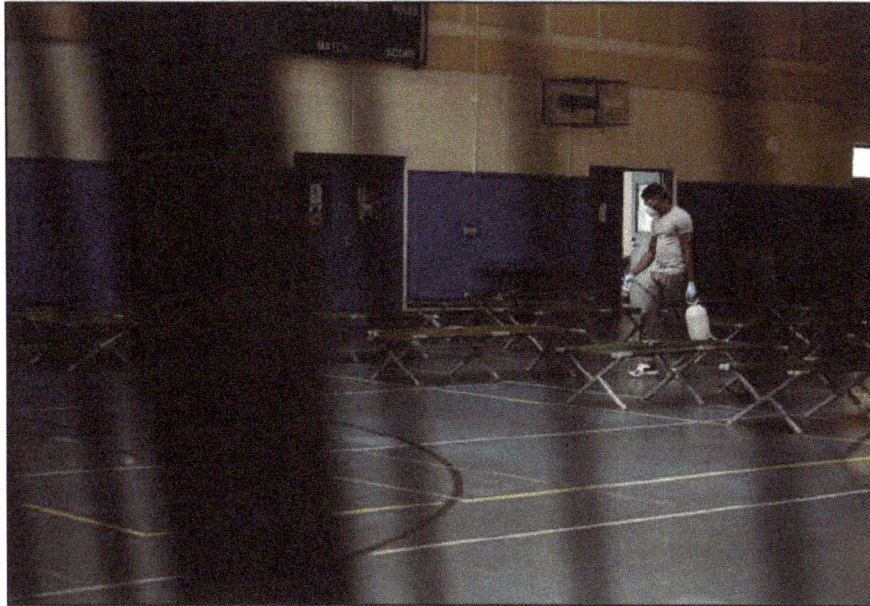

Figure 12:  Gym Cot Setup

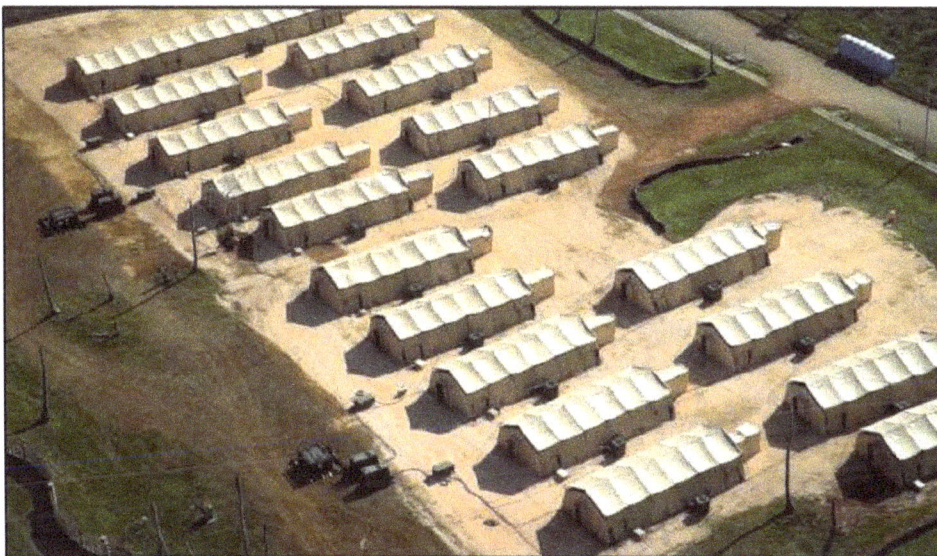

Figure 13:  Guam Expeditionary Medical Facility (EMF)

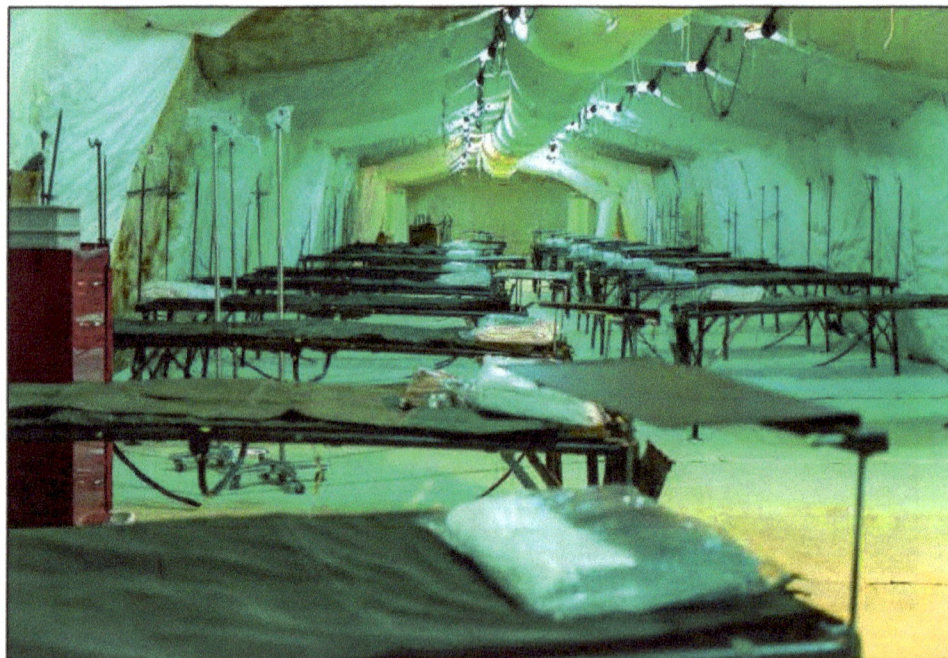

*Figure 14:  Guam EMF*

When the Government of Guam issued a state of public health emergency on March 14[th], Naval Base Guam set Health Protection Condition Level (HPCON) C+.  This HPCON significantly limited personnel on and transit within the base.  Additionally, the pier area around TR had been designated a Force Health Protection Boundary (FHPB), restricting movement for TR's Sailors off the pier.

Delays in Disembarking Crew

C7F said he believed that the TR CO and CSG-9 were resisting sending the crew ashore because available facilities were not fully CDC compliant.[200]  Some of the spaces available are pictured in Figures 15 and 16 below.

---

[200] C7F COS Statement dtd 21 May 20

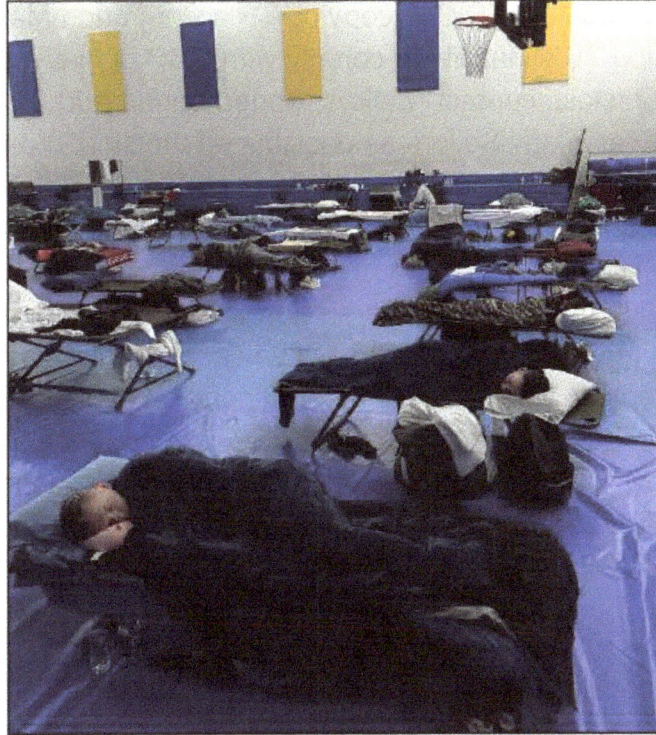

Figure 15: USS Theodore Roosevelt (CVN 71) Sailors quarantined in gym (US Navy Photo)

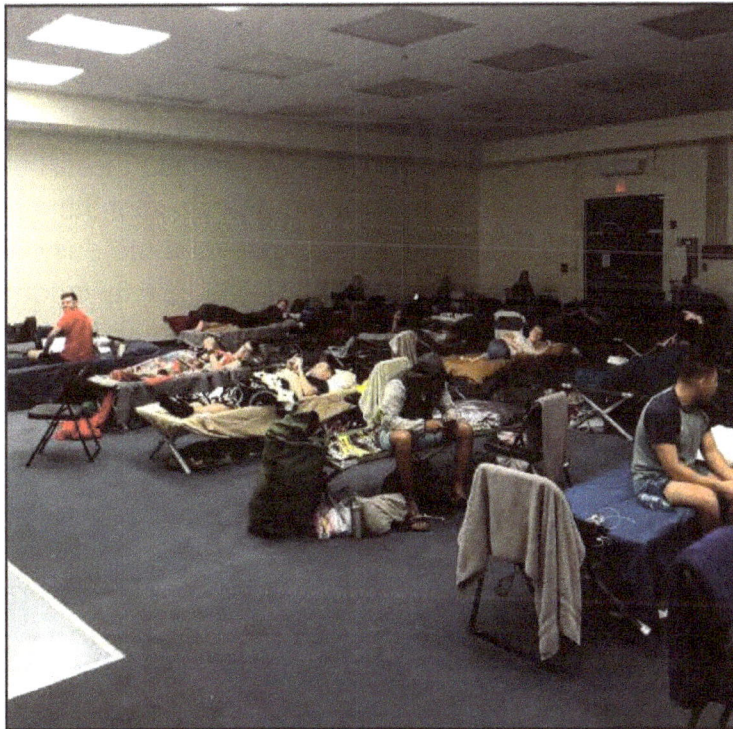

Figure 16: USS Theodore Roosevelt (CVN 71) Sailors quarantined in facility on Guam (US Navy Photo)

On March 28th, TR XO emailed TR CO, copying TR's Command Master Chief (CMC) and TR SMO, regarding TR's inability to comply with CDC or Navy guidelines aboard the ship. Estimates of "close contact" Sailors ranged from 1,400-2,000. TR XO recommended moving as many Sailors as possible off the ship into lodging. TR XO stood up the Emergency Command Center (ECC) onboard the TR and placed the Combat Direction Center Officer (CDCO) in charge on the first full day pierside in Guam (March 28th). TR XO suggested that the ECC data demonstrated the ship's segregated berthing plan was making the rate of transmission worse.[201] According to email updates sent to CCSG-9 from the TR SMO, tested positive cases were 44 at midday on March 28th,[202] 46 in the evening of March 28th,[203] 50 at midday on March 29th,[204] and 53 in the evening of March 29th.[205] The SMO stated to CCSG-9 in an email, "we have lost" against COVID-19 on TR.[206] This conclusion was incorrect, as those in segregated berthing had been placed there due to close contact tracing, and had a higher likelihood of showing symptoms. A higher rate of COVID cases in quarantine areas should have been expected.

Prior to the hotels becoming available, the testing requirement for Sailors going ashore was not completely understood by TR CO, TR XO, and TR SMO. In his interview statement, the C7F COS stated that 100 percent testing was not required and that message was clearly communicated, however, on March 28th, he told the CSG-9 COS that TR was not following "protocol" because Sailors were going into quarantine without batch tests to determine if the virus was present.[207] In their interview statements, TR CO stated that testing was required, XO stated that 100 percent testing was not being conducted, and TR SMO stated that he was confused over testing requirements but did not agree with 100 percent testing.[208] Supervisors, to include the TR CO and CCSG-9, were unaware of this confusion and the associated delays. Contributing to this, the TR SMO did not consistently attend or send a representative to the daily C7F medical synchronization meetings because the medical staff was heavily loaded with patient care and testing.[209] As a result, this issue was never brought to the attention of C7F for resolution until the preliminary inquiry identified it.

By March 29th, the testing rates for TR were up to 120 per day and there were 4,389 crew remaining to be tested, which would take 37 more days at that rate.[210] The ship

[201] TR XO Statement dtd 16 May 20
[202] Email – TR SMO to CCSG-9 – COVID-19 update 28 March - Mid-day update dtd 28 Mar 20
[203] Email – TR SMO to CCSG-9 – RE COVID -19 update 29 March – Evening update dtd 28 Mar 20
[204] Email – TR SMO to CCSG-9 – COVID-19 update 29 March - Mid-day update 29 Mar 20
[205] Email – TR SMO to CCSG-9 – COVID-19 update 29 March - Evening update dtd 29 Mar 20
[206] Email - TR SMO to C7F and CPF Surgeons – Reality dtd 28 Mar 20
[207] Email (SIPR) – COS C7F to COS CSG-9 – Triage and procedure dtd 28 Mar 20
[208] C7F COS Statement dtd 21 May 20; Crozier, B. CAPT Statement dtd 15 May 20; TR XO Statement dtd 16 May 20; TR SMO Statement dtd 17 May 20
[209] CPF Surgeon Statement dtd 19 May 20
[210] Email (SIPR) – C7F COS – Numbers dtd 29 Mar 20

was down to the last 100 test swabs. More swabs were inbound, but not expected to be delivered until after April 2nd.


## Alternate Housing Options Discussed

During planning sessions on March 27th, III MEF and C7F refined Okinawa's available capacity to approximately 3,000 rooms. Atsugi was also expected to have 400-600 rooms. However, the C7F planning diagram[211] was distributed showing rooms on Guam as available that were not yet ready. Further, rooms on Okinawa were listed as "White Beach: 5,700 and Commander, Fleet Activity Okinawa (CFAO): 0." Although CFAO owns White Beach, III MEF billeting is not located at White Beach (see Figure 17). C7F had arranged for III MEF to vacate their barracks in Okinawa located at MCAS Futenma, MCB Butler and outlying camps. This would have made 5,700 rooms available on the Marine Corps bases, not White Beach that CFAO had cognizance over. The TR CO and CSG-9 Warfare Commanders stated that they were unaware of this intended movement of III MEF.

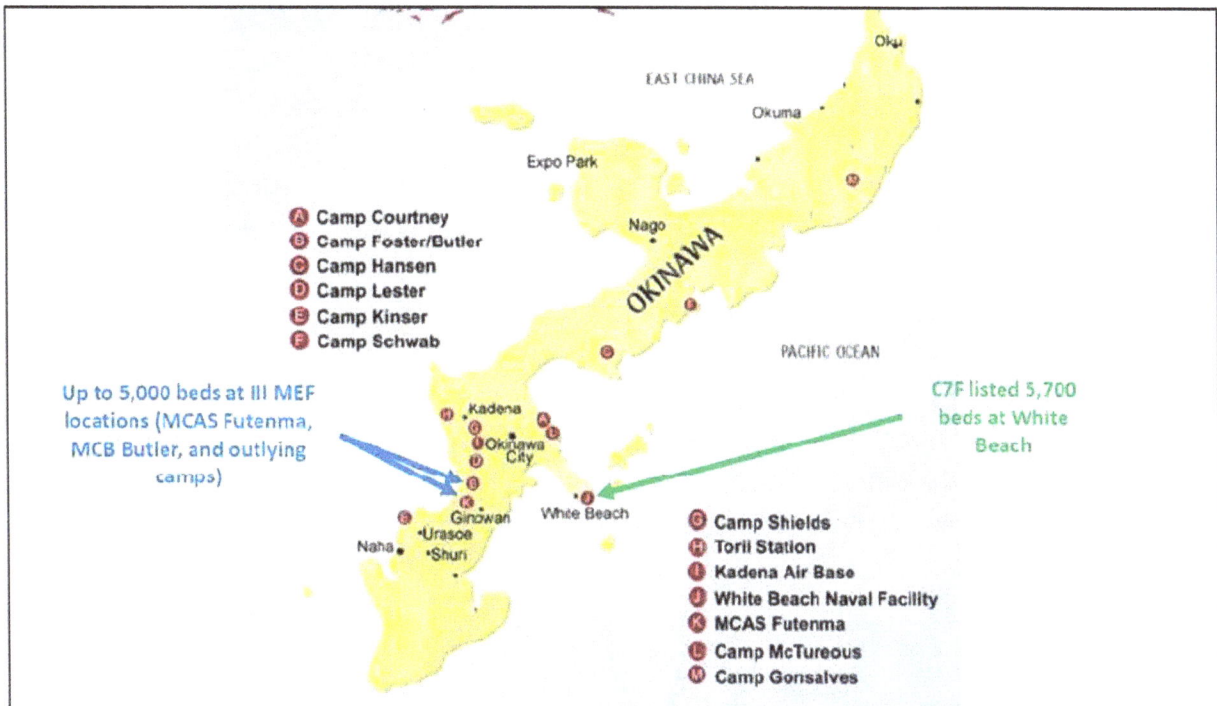

Figure 17. Location of beds in Okinawa.

---

[211] (S) C7F TR COVID Placemat 29 Mar - DRAFT

On March 28th, CCSG-9 and TR were tasked to develop plans to airlift crew members to Okinawa. After hours of work towards this task, the TR CO emailed an acquaintance, a Navy Captain at Kadena Air Force Base on Okinawa, to confirm the availability of appropriate and sufficient berthing and was told there were insufficient bunks available.[212] The TR CO discussed this with the TR XO and senior Warfare Commanders. They said they believed the C7F staff had wasted their time on a non-viable COA. The TR CO did not attempt to verify the accuracy of this information up the chain of command.[213] The same day, initial discussions about increasing capacity via hotels occurred between CJRM and his Chief of Staff.[214]

CJRM began consulting with the Government of Guam on March 28th[215] to obtain hotel rooms, independent and without any knowledge of the ship's expectations. While the TR CO and CSG-9 Warfare Commanders indicated they were not fully aware of the details regarding the Guam hotel COA,[216] CCSG-9 was aware of ongoing efforts by higher headquarters to negotiate for the use of hotels on Guam. TR CO was also aware that higher headquarters were working toward securing hotels on Guam.[217]

From the onset of the first MEDEVAC flights on March 25th[218] from TR, JRM and TR received support from the people and Government of Guam led by Governor Leon Guerrero. Following CJRM's notifications of the first three MEDEVAC patients on March 25th and 21 more COVID-positive patients on March 26th, communications between JRM and the Government of Guam significantly increased.[219]

Following the initial CJRM calls on March 28th, during which the Governor pledged her assistance saying that "we (Guam) need to support the people who defend us. This is the humanitarian thing to do."[220] JRM staff quickly began identifying the scope and requirements for support. The Governor's COS provided an initial referral to the President of the Guam Hotel and Restaurant Association (GHRA) on March 29th. The detailed, immediate planning was led by COS, JRM and the President of GHRA, in conjunction with TR leadership between March 30th and April 1st. As this delicate coordination was taking place, the President of the GHRA passed along a string of emails where an unknown person from the TR was looking to book hundreds of rooms

---

[212] Crozier, B. CAPT Statement dtd 15 May 20; TR XO Statement dtd 16 May 20
[213] CCSG-9 Statement dtd 15 May 20; Crozier, B. CAPT Statement dtd 15 May 20; TR XO Statement dtd 16 May 20
[214] Email - CJRM – Follow Up to 13 May 20 Phone Call
[215] Email - CJRM – Follow Up to 13 May 20 Phone Call; C7F COS statement dtd 21 May 20
[216] Crozier, B. CAPT Statement dtd 15 May 20; CVW-11 CAG Statement dtd 19 May 20; CDS-23 Statement dtd 19 May 20; CSG-9 COS Statement dtd 18 May 20
[217] C7F Statement dtd 18 May 20
[218] Email – TR SMO to CCSG-9 – COVID-19 update 25 Mar - End of Day testing results dtd 25 Mar 20
[219] Email - CJRM – Follow Up to 13 May 20 Phone Call
[220] Email - CJRM – Follow Up to 13 May 20 Phone Call

in Guam for the TR.[221] When informed of this, TR XO emailed all leadership on TR to ask personnel to stop, as this was "counterproductive" as Guam political leaders were "under tremendous pressure from their constituents to contain [the TR COVID cases] to the base" and noted that currently there was "little local support for moving" TR Sailors into hotels on the island.[222] After the initial concept of operations was developed and GHRA identified the first hotels, a unified "walkthrough" of partner hotels was arranged on April 1st and 2nd at various sites.[223]

On March 29th, TR had 53 positive cases with at least seven showing symptoms.[224] CPF directed that no Navy personnel leave Guam until he personally reviewed and approved that plan, effectively putting a hold on the Okinawa COA.[225] The TR SMO assessed that up to half of the ship was a close contact making the continued use of the quarantine areas aboard as ineffective.[226] The TR XO considered that conditions in the aft quarantine area were creating "human suffering" and that the large number of Sailors in the aft quarantine area was unmanageable.[227]

The same day, with an estimated total exceeding 1,000 Sailors in quarantine, the TR CO released these Sailors in aft quarantine based on the recommendation of the TR SMO and TR XO.[228] Additionally, there were large numbers of Sailors in quarantine and the TR XO considered the spaces to which they were confined to be very crowded.[229] The TR CO made the decision without consulting CCSG-9 but later informed him of his decision.[230] The CO, NBG and C7F COS believed that if they could not achieve more social distancing ashore, more Sailors would develop the virus.[231] C7F and CPF were neither informed nor consulted on this critical decision.[232]

The CSG-9 Warfare Commanders, TR CO and TR XO developed an information paper which would later inform a COA development discussion with CCSG-9.[233]

The Warfare Commanders' email and attached information paper stated that testing cannot determine who does not have the virus, it can only confirm who does, and further stressed that TR could not become a "clean" ship leveraging testing alone.

[221] Email – TR PAO to JRM PAO et al. – RE: IMMEDIATE AWARENESS" >> Fwd: 400 Rooms checking in ASAP dtd 31 Mar 20
[222] Email - TR XO - Hotel Room inquires dtd 31 Mar 0202
[223] Email - CJRM – Follow Up to 13 May 20 Phone Call
[224] Email – TR SMO to CCSG-9 – COVID-19 update 29 March - Evening update dtd 29 Mar 20
[225] Email (SIPR) – CPF to C7F – RE (S) C7F COVID-19 Update 29 Mar CORRECT COPY!!! dtd 29 Mar 20
[226] TR SMO Statement dtd 17 May 20
[227] TR XO Statement dtd 16 May 20
[228] Crozier, B. CAPT Statement dtd 15 May 20; TR XO Statement dtd 16 May 20
[229] TR XO Statement dtd 16 May 20; Crozier, B. CAPT Statement dtd 15 May 20
[230] CCSG-9 Statement dtd 15 May 20; Crozier, B. CAPT Statement dtd 15 May 20
[231] Email (SIPR) - NBG CO to C7F COS - Quarantine - Social Distancing - getting to 4,000 dtd 29 Mar 20
[232] CPF Surgeon Statement dtd 19 May 20, C7F Statement dtd 18 May 20
[233] Crozier, B. CAPT Statement dtd 15 May 20; TR XO Statement dtd 16 May 20; CVW-11 CAG Statement dtd 19 May 20; CDS-23 Statement dtd 19 May 20

Applying their interpretation of lessons learned from the cruise ship Diamond Princess to the TR situation, the paper concluded that 1) 500 additional infections occurred due to quarantine aboard versus isolation ashore and 2) 47 percent of positives were initially asymptomatic. By this reasoning, Sailors initially thought to be safe, were not. The letter stated the absence of symptoms did not indicate lack of infection much like negative test results do not indicate lack of infection. This paper, which the CVW-11 CAG emailed to CCSG-9 on March 29[th], would later form the basis of the CO's letter.

CCSG-9 concurred with the recommendation and proposed the Guam hotel COA to C7F the next day (March 30[th]), and while acknowledging the request and knowing that CCSG-9 was aware of ongoing negotiations for the hotel rooms, C7F directed him to continue to focus on Okinawa as the primary COA. Bringing TR to NBG had been predicated by a guarantee from CPF to the Government of Guam that no support would be required from them.[234] C7F did not view the temporary facilities as inadequate as they were a short-term improvement over shipboard conditions that would provide a bridge to a longer-term solution.[235] The longer-term solution would be Okinawa or Guam hotels.

Ultimately, on March 29[th], CPF was not ready to approve C7F's plan for moving the TR crew to Okinawa based on the risk of accelerating infection spread on the aircraft during the 9-hour flight to that island, and complications with the government of Japan.[236] At the time, there were 1,167 beds available on Guam, of which 535 were occupied.[237]

As mentioned earlier, prior to TR's arrival in Guam, CSG-9 COS emailed C7F COS to relay the recommendation from TR CO and TR SMO that 4,000 hotel rooms should be obtained in Guam.[238] C7F, CCSG-9, CJRM and TR all understood the requirement for 4,000 beds, with no discussion of the beds being CDC compliant (i.e., one bed and one head per room).

Days Leading to Relief of TR CO

By this point, the TR CO, TR XO and CSG-9 Warfare Commanders were frustrated. They felt they had been distracted by numerous RFIs from higher headquarters, and by working COAs that they did not believe in, and that in the end, they were going to be made to stay in the makeshift berthing on Guam, long-term, which they viewed as

[234] UPDATED: USS Theodore Roosevelt Quarantines Sailors on Guam as Coronavirus Outbreak Spreads, *USNI News* (26 Mar 20)
[235] C7F Statement dtd 18 May 20
[236] Email (SIPR) – CPF to C7F – Evening Ops Update and COVID 29 Mar dtd 29 Mar 20
[237] Email - CJRM – Follow Up to 13 May 20 Phone Call
[238] Email (SIPR) – CSG-9 COS to C7F COS – (U) HOTEL OPTION dtd 25 Mar 20

worse than the ship. Further, they considered that available rooms on Okinawa never existed, and that the whole event had been a distraction. This was compounded by the continued increase in number of COVID-19 positive Sailors and the worst-case narrative of TR fatalities that continued to be pressed forward by the TR SMO and championed by key TR and CSG-9 leadership.

None of these leaders took action to openly communicate these concerns directly with C7F, VADM Merz, although they had a voice at the daily briefs.

Believing that the C7F staff was not seriously entertaining or working towards obtaining CDC compliant hotel rooms in Guam for crew isolation and quarantine, the TR CO and TR SMO elected to bypass their chains of command, and took parallel actions to take matters into their own hands, described in Chapter 4 below.

On March 28th, a JRM COS telephone call with the Governor of Guam COS revealed positive indications on the hotel option, and that the Governor required a formal request from CPF or INDOPACOM.[239] That same day, the TR SMO wrote an email to C7F and PACFLT Surgeons stating the need to get 4,500 personnel into individual berthing with single heads.[240] On March 31st, with 1,450 Sailors aboard TR in quarantine or isolation, CPF formally requested Guam hotel options and negotiations commenced for an undetermined number of hotel rooms.[241] Also that day, the TR SMO sent an email to the Navy Surgeon General, restating the need to get at least 4,500 personnel off the ship and into single berthing.[242]

NBG, C7F, and TR agreed to the egress strategy and its prioritization of categories of Sailors. Dissatisfied with the pace of egress, C7F repeatedly prompted CCSG-9 for TR's plan to utilize the isolation and quarantine quarters available. With no plan in hand four days after the ship's arrival, and with hundreds of temporary quarantine bunks remaining unused, C7F issued "C7F TASKORD for Recovery of USS Theodore Roosevelt from COVID-19 Infection" on April 1st, formally requiring development of this plan, the same day the San Francisco Chronicle published a copy of the TR CO's memo.

On April 2nd, the TR CO sent letters to family members regarding the memo stating, "It was never my intention to have the letter made public." The CO's letter to the families stated that every Sailor would be tested for COVID-19 and those with negative test results would be moved to individual rooms off base for 14 days, while those who tested

---

[239] C7F Statement dtd 18 May 20; Email - CJRM – Follow Up to 13 May 20 Phone Call
[240] Email - TR SMO - Reality dtd 28 Mar 20
[241] C7F Statement dtd 18 May 20
[242] Email – TR SMO to Navy Surgeon General – Situation on the Ground dtd 30 Mar 20

positive would be housed on base in individual rooms. The letter indicated that some Sailors would remain aboard to clean the ship before moving off to complete their 14-day isolation.

TR Sailors began occupying Guam hotels on the morning of April 2nd. Of the 2,343 isolation and quarantine beds available on NBG, 1,283 remained vacant when the CO was relieved later that day.[243]

Following the A-SN's April 2nd (D.C. date) public announcement of his direction to relieve TR CO, CCSG-9 relieved the TR CO on April 3rd (Guam date). Prior to the former TR CO's departure, TR XO made notification to TR heads of department (HODs) of the former CO's departure from the ship.[244] As former TR CO departed the ship through the hangar bay and via the officer's brow to the pier, hundreds of Sailors gathered to witness the former CO's departure. In multiple open-source videos, the Sailors are seen amassing and then cheering and chanting his name with only a small number wearing masks and with no social distancing (see Figure 18 below). Most of the videos taken and then shared on social media, online video sharing sites, and with news outlets, were taken by Sailors.

---

[243] C7F Statement dtd 18 May 20; Email - CJRM – Follow Up to 13 May 20 Phone Call
[244] CCSG-9 Statement dtd 15 May 20

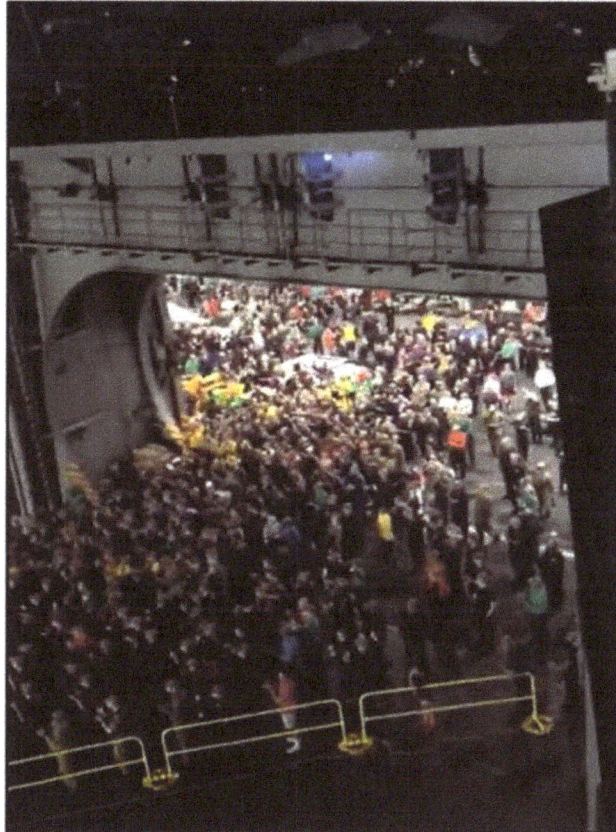

*Figure 18. TR crew cheers former TR CO as he departs the ship after being relieved of command on April 3, 2020 (https://nypost.com/2020/04/03/capt-brett-crozier-gets-dramatic-send-off-from-sailors/)*

In his testimony to the investigation team, CCSG-9 recalled the former TR CO's departure and his reaction to the event. He stated that when he witnessed the videos, he immediately contacted TR XO and asked for an explanation to which the TR XO stated that he had alerted the HODs of the former TR CO's departure but had no reply to CCSG-9 regarding the ensuing mass of Sailors in close proximity in the hangar bay still not practicing social distancing. CCSG-9 further stated that he assessed the crew had an understanding of COVID-19 at the time but did not appreciate the seriousness.[245] In his testimony to the investigative team, C7F recounted the significant concerns he had following his viewing of the videos and restated his comment to the Sailors aboard TR that "our job just got a lot harder."[246]

---

[245] CCSG-9 Statement dtd 15 May 20
[246] C7F Statement dtd 18 May 20

## Chapter 4 – Development of and Response to USS Theodore Roosevelt (CVN 71) Commanding Officer Letter of March 30, 2020

This chapter addresses the preparation and email delivery of the former commanding officer's letter dated March 30, 2020, further handling of that email, and response to the email and letter by the chain of command. This chapter refers to transcripts and summaries of public statements made by Department of the Navy officials related to the relief of the former commanding officer.

Preparations for Arrival in Guam

Prior to TR's arrival on March 27[th], the CO, NBG and staff addressed berthing arrangements needed for COVID patients from TR. Upon TR's arrival in Guam, TR CO requested to CO, NBG berthing arrangements for the ship's crew that centered upon fully meeting the requirements of CDC Guidance and Navy guidance[247] were prioritized. From March 25[th] onward, TR and CCSG-9 recommended 4,000 beds as the preferred COA, using hotels in Guam as well as potentially alternate locations including Okinawa and Atsugi.[248]

NBG provided a laydown of alternative berthing arrangements prior to arrival and during the port visit that met many but not all of the parameters TR CO and TR XO believed Navy guidance required.[249] The ship did not have a means of tracking where the crew members were going until the TR XO activated the Emergency Command Center (ECC) on March 28[th] to centralize requests and information flow. The ECC operated out of the TR XO conference room principally to answer RFIs.[250]

Warfare Commanders White Paper for CCSG-9

The TR CO, TR XO and TR SMO all stated they collectively believed that by TR's fourth day in Guam there were no clear plans to move 4,000 personnel off the ship into isolation and quarantine in CDC compliant facilities in which each person would have their own room and bathroom and be supplied with appropriate food, ventilation and air conditioning.

---

[247] NAVADMIN 083/20 Restriction of Movement (ROM) Guidance dtd 23 Mar 20
[248] Email (SIPR) – CSG-9 COS to C7F COS – (U) HOTEL OPTION dtd 25 Mar 20
[249] The TR CO and TR XO interviews cite NAVADMIN 083/20: "For transient personnel and those residing in close quarters such as unaccompanied housing or ships, temporary lodging meeting CDC guidance of separate sleeping and bathroom facilities shall be arranged, when available"
[250] TR XO Statement dtd 16 May 20; CDCO Statement dtd 18 May 20 (digitally signed)

On March 29[th], the CVW-11 CAG sent a white paper presenting a COVID-19 analysis and suggested COAs to CCSG-9.  The white paper was produced in collaboration with Warfare Commanders and TR senior leadership.  The goal was to provide options for CCSG-9 to bring to C7F to spur action toward a safer situation for the crew of TR.  After receiving the white paper, CCSG-9 directed the Warfare Commanders to distill it into four executable COAs.  CVW-11 CAG sent the "Warfare Commander's Courses of Action"[251] white paper which outlined the following possible avenues to address the growing outbreak on the ship:

1.  4,500 Sailor individual isolation; 500 remain to run ship; swap & deploy

2.  2,500 in individual isolation / 2,500 on board TR and in group berthing off-ship

3.  Status Quo – group berthing off-ship using available NBG facilities

4.  Immediately get underway

CVW-11 CAG stated that the COAs were designed to minimize the number of Sailors exposed to COVID-19 and regain warfighting readiness as soon as possible.  The Warfare Commanders met with CCSG-9 to discuss the options available to combat the growing crisis.  CCSG-9 listened to the counsel of his subordinates before explaining that there was a desire to keep the solution to the problem within Navy channels and that the hotel issue needed to be resolved with the Governor of Guam.  CVW-11 CAG stated that the paper and subsequent COA development prompted CCSG-9 to keep pressing C7F for solutions to individual isolation challenges.[252]

The CSG-9 COS stated he believed the Warfare Commanders provided CCSG-9 with the white paper because they were frustrated with the way ahead and wanted CCSG-9 to "jump the chain of command" to CPF for additional emphasis.[253]

CCSG-9 requested 4,000 CDC compliant rooms on March 25[th] with higher headquarters.[254]  However, according to CCSG-9, the feedback he received was that the Guam hotels were really not an option because the A-SN had said publicly that the U.S. Government would not use the resources of Guam.[255]  Specifically, A-SN stated during a press conference on March 26[th] that, "[t]he ship [TR] is pulling into Guam; it will be pierside, no one on the crew will be allowed to leave anywhere into Guam other than

---

[251] Email - CVW-11 CAG – Four COAs – WARFARE COMMANDER DEVELOPED PROs & CONs / RISK TO MISSION & RISK TO FORCE dtd 29 Mar 20
[252] CVW-11 CAG Statement dtd 19 May 20
[253] CSG-9 COS Statement dtd 18 May 20
[254] CCSG-9 Statement dtd 15 May 20
[255] CCSG-9 Statement dtd 15 May 20

on pierside. And we are already starting the process of testing 100 percent of the crew to ensure that we've got that contained."[256] Despite this public statement from A-SN, CCSG-9 did not believe using the local resources of Guam was completely off the table.[257] However, C7F and CPF were, in fact sensitive to making the request, as the Navy had promised to not impose upon the Government of Guam, who was dealing with its own public health emergency.[258] In addition, on the morning of March 30th, CCSG-9 recommended to C7F (via video-teleconference) removal of 4,500 Sailors to individual isolation rooms based on both the white paper and COAs in development by the Warfare Commanders. C7F acknowledged the recommendation but directed to continue batch testing, identification of "clean" groups, and development of plan to get a "clean" ship.[259]

TR CO stated that he was unaware of any promises the U.S. Government had made to Guam about the use of local resources to aid in the care of Navy Sailors.[260] He did, however, acknowledge that the A-SN's COS had understood they needed more cots on base and attributed the acceleration of that delivery to his interaction. Subsequent information provided by A-SN's COS indicated that he did not specifically direct any additional resources as he was informed CPF and TR's chain of command were addressing all needed support.[261]

CVW-11 CAG outlined that while the NBG facilities were appreciated, they were not sufficiently isolating personnel per the TR SMO's guidance. He stated they "knew that securing hotels for the entire TR crew was impractical upon arrival and were careful to ask for isolation, not specifically hotel rooms."[262]

## Development of the TR CO Letter and Email

The TR XO indicated that the TR CO's letter was an abridged version of the white paper to which all CSG-9 Warfare Commanders had contributed. The TR XO said CCSG-9 and C7F were concerned why more available berthing on Guam was not occupied. He explained the growing sense of frustration present on board as they (TR CO, TR XO and Warfare Commanders) started to hear and note positive tests of Sailors in the open

---

[256] Transcript: Marine Corps Officials Hold a Defense Department News Briefing on COVID-19 Efforts dtd 26 Mar 20 https://www.defense.gov/Newsroom/Transcripts/Transcript/Article/2127585/marine-corps-officials-hold-a-defense-department-news-briefing-on-covid-19-effo/
[257] CCSG-9 Statement dtd 15 May 20
[258] CPF Statement dtd 17 May 20; C7F Statement dtd 18 May 20; Email - CJRM – Follow Up to 13 May 20 Phone Call
[259] CVW-11 CAG Statement dtd 19 May 20
[260] Crozier, B. CAPT Statement dtd 15 May 20
[261] Email - A-SN COS to DNS – RE: Support Requirements dtd 30 Mar 20
[262] CVW-11 CAG Statement dtd 19 May 20

bay gym settings (the open bay areas were notionally for "clean crew" who would make up critical watchstanders needed to get the ship underway). He further discussed the large number of Sailors requiring care and feeding, stating that inconsistent meal service and availability of sanitary facilities led to Sailor complaints on social media and to families in San Diego. Additionally, the TR XO stated that he was frustrated with discussion over COAs that could not fully comply with NAVADMIN guidance.[263]

While the TR CO and TR XO waited for a possible phone call they believed would be coming from the CNO[264] on the morning of March 30th, the TR CO asked TR XO to shorten and simplify the much longer Warfare Commanders' information paper. The investigation found that the CNO had not planned to call the TR CO. The anticipated call was confused with another request from the CNO's Battle Watch Captain (BWC) calling TR to ask if the previous A-SN COS call had been completed.[265] The TR XO stressed that neither he nor TR CO knew at this time of any momentum or desire to obtain individual isolation rooms for Sailors on Guam (i.e., the hotel options). The TR XO sat at the large table in the TR CO's In-Port Cabin and worked on this project with pen and ink. The TR XO did not know to whom the TR CO meant to address the letter, so he it left that section blank. The TR CO simultaneously composed the email cover letter. The TR XO presented his notes to the TR CO and then used the Ship's Secretary's computer to turn the notes into a four page memo (CO's Letter). The TR CO made edits to the opening and closing paragraphs while the TR XO proof-read the email the TR CO had written. Once the TR CO was satisfied with both documents, he signed and scanned the four page memo, attached it to his email and sent it to CPF, CNAP and CCSG-9. The TR XO estimated both documents were written in two to three hours. The only individuals involved in drafting those documents were the TR CO and TR XO with administrative support from the Ship's Secretary.[266]

The TR CO received calls and emails from A-SN's COS on March 30th at 0525 and the evening of March 30th to address a visit by the Secretary on April 1st and voice support for, as well as assistance to, TR. CPF had also called the TR CO on March 29th to notify him that A-SN would be calling (which ended up being the A-SN COS). CPF asked if any additional assistance was required, and the TR CO indicated he was getting what he needed.[267] The TR CO did not specify an immediate need for 4,000

---

[263] TR XO Statement dtd 16 May 20; Email - TR XO to TR CO - Memo for Record - Failure to comply with NAVADMIN 083_20 dtd 28 Mar 20

[264] Email - CNO Former EA to TR CI Senior Legal Advisor – TR Investigation dtd 20 May 20 (noting CNO was not requested, nor did he intend, to contact TR CO by phone directly at any time relevant to this investigation instead trusting "the leadership in [the TR] Chain of Command to discuss the immediate issues of the ship with" the TR CO).

[265] Email CNO ABWC PTGN to BWC PTGN RE: Hot RFI.THEODORE ROOSEVELT RFI dtd 30 Mar 20; email CNO EA to BWC PTGN FW: TR dtd 29 Mar 20; Email - CNO Former EA to TR CI Senior Legal Advisor – TR Investigation dtd 20 May 20

[266] TR XO Statement dtd 16 May 20; TR RO Statement dtd 18 May 20; CVW-11 CAG Statement dtd 19 May 20

[267] CPF Statement dtd 17 May 20

beds fully in compliance with CDC and Navy guidelines in those conversations and did not specify that the current plans were not acceptable.[268]

On March 30[th] at 1348, the TR CO sent an email containing the letter drafted by TR XO to ten recipients:  addressed to CPF, CNAP, CSG-9, and copied to CVW-11 CAG, TR XO, CVW-11 Deputy CAG, CDS 23, TR SMO, CPF COS, and CNAP COS.

In the attached paper ("Request for Assistance in Response to COVID-19 Pandemic," dated March 30[th]), the TR CO specifically requested "all available resources to find NAVADMIN and CDC compliant quarantine rooms for my entire crew as soon as possible."[269]  This was the only specific resource request outlined and did not specify what command was responsible for delivery of these rooms nor did it indicate how many rooms or beds required, were currently available and in use.  He stated that his letter "was designed to bring a sense of urgency to what we thought was a growing tragedy."[270]  He "wanted to stop the administrative bureaucracy" and "bring focus back to what we thought was the best course of action to get people off the ship."[271]

The TR CO used unclassified email to send the email and letter instead of a classified network.  In addition, he anticipated that the style and method would be more urgent and quicker to read on mobile devices and that he wanted a timely response.[272]  TR CO mentioned that the majority of work and updates regarding the ship was conducted on the unclassified network (daily COVID-19 reports on the number of positive cases).  He stated that he did not foresee a leak to the press nor did he anticipate any difficulties the letter would generate with the negotiations with the Governor of Guam.

One key aspect of the TR CO's letter attached to the email is the sense of urgency tied the consequences of inaction.  "Sailors do not need to die" and "If we do not act now, we are failing to properly take care of our most trusted asset – our Sailors" reflect the underlying theme of both the email and letter.[273]

Reactor Department Email

The TR Reactor Officer (RO) expressed concern about the ability to keep the Reactor Department watch supervisors safely isolated so they could perform their jobs as

[268] Crozier, B. CAPT Statement dtd 15 May 20; CPF Statement dtd 17 May 20
[269] TR CO Email and Ltr - Request for Assistance in Response to COVID-19 Pandemic dtd 30 Mar 20
[270] Crozier, B. CAPT Statement dtd 15 May 20
[271] Crozier, B. CAPT Statement dtd 15 May 20
[272] Crozier, B. CAPT Statement dtd 15 May 20
[273] TR CO Email and Ltr - Request for Assistance in Response to COVID-19 Pandemic dtd 30 Mar 20

required. The TR RO's Sailors were going to the gym. This was a problem because the gym was getting one or two positive hits a day for COVID. The TR RO went to talk to the TR CO who showed her the letter that he and the TR XO were drafting with some assistance from the Ship's Secretary. The TR RO mentioned that she had a very good relationship with Naval Reactors (NR) and stressed that as an RO she may speak to the Admiral directly with any concerns. On March 26th, the TR RO sent an email to CNAP and NR via the classified network that outlined the current situation and way ahead for operations.[274] On March 30th, after observing that several Sailors were testing positive in the gyms (ostensibly a segregated zone for "clean" COVID-negative critical watchstanders), she became concerned about the lodging situation of her Sailors and was worried about her ability to re-man the department in a timely manner. After consulting with TR CO and seeing the email and memo that TR XO and TR CO were drafting, she drafted a classified email which the TR CO subsequently sent to CNAP on March 30th at 1938 with the subject line: "COVID-19 Pandemic – TR request for assistance."[275] This email was very similar to the chain of command email and voiced concerns about manning watch teams and outlined the need to house Sailors "off ship in true isolation rooms with separate bathroom facilities." However, not enough time would have passed for Sailors who tested positive or were showing symptoms while being assigned to common areas like a gym to have actually become infected while assigned there; instead, given the timing, any Sailors showing symptoms at this time would have had to become infected earlier while aboard the ship. To the degree anyone may have believed that Sailors had become infected in such a common area, their analysis was actually flawed due to the timing.

Medical Department Letter

On March 28th, the TR SMO sent an email to the CPF, C7F and CNAP Surgeons stating, "We have lost," and declaring the "'quarantine' measures on the ship are a sham."[276] The TR SMO also noted that TR was "failing to comply with any sort of [testing guidelines] . . . or guidelines on quarantine" and needed "to implement appropriate quarantine measures . . . which will involve getting 4,500 people off the ship into individual berthing with single heads."[277] The TR SMO also communicated to CCSG-9 his opinions that the testing required to allow Sailors to move ashore was "a waste of time." The TR SMO felt that testing would not prove whether or not a Sailor

---

[274] Email (SIPR) – TR RO to NR, CNAP RO – FW: CVN-71 COVID-19 Roll Up and Way Ahead dtd 26 Mar 20
[275] Email (SIPR) – TR CO to CNAP RO – (C) COVID-19 Pandemic – TR Request for Assistance dtd 30 Mar 20
[276] Email - TR SMO to C7F and CPF Surgeons – Reality dtd 28 Mar 20
[277] Email - TR SMO to C7F and CPF Surgeons – Reality dtd 28 Mar 20

had the virus. He did not believe that if an individual "pops negative" it did not mean that the person was "clean." He believed it to be "a waste of his resources and time to test everyone on the ship" and repeated to CCSG-9 that "you can't test your way out of this virus."[278]

The TR SMO also sent an email to the Surgeon General of the Navy on March 31st, copying the CPF and C7F Surgeons along with a small group of other senior leaders in Navy medicine. The TR SMO's email contained a letter signed by the TR SMO and four other members of the medical staff aboard.[279] This letter did not outline specific requests but relayed a sense of urgency about the situation aboard TR at the time and lamented the lack of action to treat Sailors in accordance with CDC and NAVADMIN 083/20 guidance. It also stressed the high likelihood of casualties and asserted they could have up to 50 deaths onboard based on their assessment of published fatality estimates at the time. Lastly the letter states, "Our intent is to submit this letter to the public to demonstrate our concerns for the safety of our patients and your Sailors."[280]

Although the TR SMO initially emailed the medical letter to eight people, the Surgeon General of the Navy and seven others, approximately three minutes later, the TR SMO further emailed the letter to over 160 additional medical community members. None of these additional addressees were in the TR operational or administrative chains of command.

The medical team presented their letter to the TR XO at a meeting where he showed them a hard copy of the TR CO's email and letter. TR XO recommended that the medical team not send their letter and not go to the press because the TR CO just talked to leadership. He told them, "not to send the letter and that it was not helpful, and the tone was unprofessional and overly combative."[281]

This letter was subsequently presented to the TR CO at a meeting with the TR SMO and other medical staff who had signed the letter. The TR CO asked the medical team not to send their letter because he had sent an email up his chain of command and "I can't tell you not to send it if you have a moral imperative – but ask you not to send it. I think my letter will address your concerns."[282]

Certain members of the Medical Department did not sign the letter. This appears to be due to concerns about potential professional repercussions. The TR Nurse, for

---

[278] CCSG-9 Statement dtd 15 May 20
[279] Email - TR SMO to Navy Surgeon General - Letter from Medical Department on USS Theodore Roosevelt dtd 31 Mar 20
[280] Medical Department letter dtd 31 Mar 20
[281] TR XO Statement dtd 16 May 20
[282] Crozier, B. CAPT Statement dtd 15 May 20

example, stated that although she agreed with the content of the letter and level of concern, she did not sign it because she was afraid it would "affect her career."[283] The letter states it is the Medical Department's "intent . . . to submit this letter to the public to demonstrate our concerns for the safety of our patients and your Sailors."[284] However, signers of the letter indicated they had no intent to release the letter publicly, but instead wanted to "generate aggressive action to move Sailors."[285]

## Chain of Command Response to the Email and Letter

The response to the TR CO's March 30th email, with his letter attached, was swift from the chain of command. CPF and CNAP responded as soon as they received the email.[286] CNAP responded thanking TR CO "for the red flare" and offered his help,[287] also looping in C7F and CJRM who were not on the initial communication from the TR CO. CPF responded to TR CO and CCSG-9 to "call [him] ASAP."[288] CPF subsequently spoke with CCSG-9 and TR CO on the speaker phone together following his receipt of the email and asked what he and TR wanted him to be doing that he was not already doing.[289] CNAP also spoke with TR CO following his email to provide mentorship and counsel and to gain insight into why he sent the email and letter.[290] TR CO confirmed the relationship with C7F and CCSG-9 were "healthy, with good communications in both directions, and plenty of communication opportunities. He also noted VADM Merz (C7F) was particularly engaged, holding multiple VTCs each day regarding the situation on the TR."[291] When he asked the TR CO why he sent the letter, the TR CO replied he "did not feel the response was moving fast enough."[292]

The TR XO stated he felt the email and letter were effective as he believed they saw "good initial movement after the email."[293] In addition to speaking with CNAP and CPF, the TR CO also received communications from CJRM offering assistance as a result of CNAP looping CJRM into the email string.[294] Specifically, CJRM responded to that email offering his, NBG, and AAFB continued support and to house what they could

---

[283] TR Nurse Statement dtd 18 May 20
[284] Medical Department letter dtd 31 Mar 20
[285] *See* e.g., TR Surgeon Statement dtd 18 May 20
[286] *See* Email - CNAP to TR CO - RE: TR request for assistance dtd 30 Mar 20; Email - CPF to TR CO and CCSG-9 - RE: TR request for assistance dtd 30 Mar 20
[287] CNAP to TR CO - RE: TR request for assistance dtd 30 Mar 20
[288] Email - CPF to TR CO and CCSG-9 - RE: TR request for assistance dtd 30 Mar 20
[289] CPF Statement dtd 17 May 20; CCSG-9 Statement dtd 15 May 20
[290] CNAP Statement dtd 13 May 20
[291] CNAP Statement dtd 13 May 20
[292] CNAP Statement dtd 13 May 20
[293] TR XO Statement dtd 16 May 20
[294] Email - CJRM – Follow Up to 13 May 20 Phone Call

"within [their] fence lines as well as transport Sailors to Anderson Air Force Base for further transfer off island should that be the COA selected."[295] CJRM also advised that he was "working the local solution to lodging outside the fence line but [was] treading lightly as that solution will be in direct opposition to the stated Navy position[296] not to place the burden on Guam's resources to solve our issue."[297]

On the other hand, CCSG-9 believed the letter did not need to be sent as all aspects of the TR-desired COA were in works and he expressed his surprise and anger upon learning that the TR CO sent the letter.[298] CCSG-9 and the TR CO discussed the letter together, with others present,[299] and also took the call from CPF about it. CPF confirmed that no new actions were taken as a result of TR CO's email and letter. He had already addressed specific requests through CJRM for hotel space in Guam. He did call the Governor of Guam on Tuesday to request rooms be made available to Sailors who were not COVID-positive.[300]

In addition, comments from CJRM, C7F and CPF also indicated the letter created significant challenges negotiating hotels with the Governor of Guam.

Publication of Letter in San Francisco Chronicle

On March 31st at 0911, a reporter from the San Francisco Chronicle contacted the Pentagon Press Operations Duty Officer via email stating he had "obtained a copy of a four-page letter sent from [TR CO] pleading for help from the U.S. Navy brass to bring equipment to allow isolated quarantines for his entire crew."[301] This media inquiry was forwarded to CPF public affairs and eventually on to TR's PAO at 1323.[302] A story from the San Francisco Chronicle, dated March 31st and entitled "Exclusive: Captain of aircraft carrier with growing coronavirus outbreak pleads for help from Navy" was posted on their website on April 1st at 0400 initially without comment from the Navy.[303] The TR CO stated he did not send the letter outside Navy channels.[304] The memorandum from

---

[295] Email - CJRM to TR CO - RE: TR request for assistance dtd 30 Mar 20
[296] UPDATED: USS Theodore Roosevelt Quarantines Sailors on Guam as Coronavirus Outbreak Spreads, *USNI News* (26 Mar 20) https://news.usni.org/2020/03/26/coronavirus-outbreak-sidelines-aircraft-carrier-uss-theodore-roosevelt
[297] Email - CJRM to TR CO - RE: TR request for assistance dtd 30 Mar 20
[298] CCSG-9 Statement dtd 15 May 20
[299] TR OPSO Statement dtd 18 May 20
[300] CPF Statement dtd 17 May 2020
[301] Email - TR PAO - dtd 31 Mar 20
[302] Email - TR PAO - dtd 31 Mar 20
[303] "Exclusive: Captain of aircraft carrier with growing coronavirus outbreak pleads for help from Navy" SF Chronicle (31 Mar 20) https://www.sfchronicle.com/bayarea/article/Exclusive-Captain-of-aircraft-carrier-with-15167883.php, accessed May 8, 2020
[304] Crozier, B. CAPT Statement dtd 15 May 20; *See also*, TR OPSO Statement dtd 18 May 20 ("I was there when the CO realized the letter was leaked; he had the news up on his computer. The CO commented that they sent the letter to his hometown paper, stating, "They're going to think I did this, but I didn't do it.")

the TR CO was included in this article without the accompanying email.  The San Francisco Chronicle article was later updated to include public comments A-SN made during an interview with CNN where he stated the Navy had "been working actually the last seven days to move those Sailors off the ship and get them into accommodations in Guam" and that they were "very engaged in this, . . . very concerned about it and . . . taking all the appropriate steps."[305]

In addition, CCSG-9 stated that the publication of the letter in the San Francisco Chronicle created additional tension between with the Navy and the Government of Guam as there had been negotiations to utilize hotels in Guam.[306]  Not only did the TR CO claim he did "not expect to see [the letter] in the open press, he also did not anticipate his letter would create difficulties with the Governor of Guam.[307]

Stories pertaining to the TR CO letter rapidly gained traction in the press and it was widely reported in print, television, and various internet news outlets.[308]

Impact on Discussions with Government of Guam

While the article did not change the Governor's support for TR, according to testimony provided by CJRM, it affected her team's opportunity to shape the public narrative for the partnership.  Eight community groups in Guam had sent a letter to the Governor of Guam urging the military to keep patients at bases until COVID-19 was eradicated.[309]

The Governor had intended to voice her support during a press conference on April 1st, in order to convey the well-managed and thoughtful civil-military response to the situation on the ship.[310]  The San Francisco Chronicle article and TR CO's memorandum changed the narrative from a measured response to a reactive one.  The

[305] "Exclusive: Captain of aircraft carrier with growing coronavirus outbreak pleads for help from Navy" SF Chronicle (31 Mar 20) https://www.sfchronicle.com/bayarea/article/Exclusive-Captain-of-aircraft-carrier-with-15167883.php, accessed May 8, 2020
[306] CCSG-9 Statement dtd 15 May 20
[307] Crozier, B. CAPT Statement dtd 15 May 20
[308] "Captain of Aircraft Carrier Pleads for Help as Virus Cases Increase Onboard" NY Times (31 Mar 20) https://www.nytimes.com/2020/03/31/us/politics/coronavirus-aircraft-carrier-theodore-roosevelt.html; "Battling an outbreak, captain of aircraft carrier asks Navy to evacuate crew" Washington Post (31 Mar 20) https://www.washingtonpost.com/national-security/battling-an-outbreak-captain-of-aircraft-carrier-asks-navy-to-evacuate-crew/2020/03/31/cfa57e1c-7363-11ea-ae50-7148009252e3_story.html; "'Sailors do not need to die,' warns captain of coronarvirus-hit U.S. aircraft carrier" Reuters (31 Mar 20) https://www.reuters.com/article/us-health-coronavirus-usa-navy/sailors-do-not-need-to-die-warns-captain-of-coronavirus-hit-u-s-aircraft-carrier-idUSKBN21I2SV; "Coronavirus: US Navy captain pleads for help over outbreak" BBC (31 Mar 20) https://www.bbc.com/news/world-us-canada-52110298; "Theodore Roosevelt captain makes urgent plea for individual quarantine sites as COVID-18 cases multiply" Military Times (31 Mar 20) https://www.militarytimes.com/news/your-navy/2020/03/31/theodore-roosevelt-captain-makes-urgent-plea-for-individual-quarantine-sites-as-covid-19-cases-multiply/
[309] "Governor: 'One Guam' approach needed to defeat virus" Pacific Daily News (31 Mar 20) https://www.guampdn.com/story/news/local/2020/03/31/governor-one-guam-approach-needed-defeat-virus/2938329001/
[310] Email - CJRM – Follow Up to 13 May 20 Phone Call

Governor's staff was concerned that the "dire situation" the TR CO described in his memorandum would result in increased public health concern among the community.[311] CJRM outlined that the concerns included the potential for more vocal opposition from anti-military activists and a negative impact on GHRA's support of the hotel COA - resulting in the loss of critical capacity to house Sailors. Ultimately, a plan to quarantine and isolate Sailors went forward, but the opportunity for a coordinated messaging initiative was lost.[312]

## Preliminary Inquiry and Relief of TR CO

On April 2nd, 2020, the CNO ordered a preliminary inquiry into the events surrounding the disembarkation of Sailors from TR in Guam, in response to cases of COVID-19.[313] While this preliminary inquiry was pending, A-SN decided to relieve the TR CO and announced his decision in a press conference with CNO where he stated that "at [his] direction, the CO of [TR] . . . was relieved by [CCSG-9]."[314] A-SN subsequently traveled to Guam where he spoke with members of the TR crew via the public address system (1MC) and met with the former CO who was at the time in quarantine as a result of his positive test for COVID-19.[315] A-SN's remarks over the 1MC were recorded by members of the crew and released to the press by means of a written transcript followed by the actual audio recording.[316] The transcript released on the internet through various news sources appears to be a true and accurate representation of A-SN's comments as heard on the recording. These remarks were also widely reported.[317]

This investigation was not directed to evaluate the A-SN's decision to fire the TR CO, and in fact, in briefing, the investigating team was counselled to specifically stay away from this topic. However, we were asked to identify statements by Department of the Navy officials on the relief of the CO that may have been in error. Where appropriate, we have identified those errors.

In A-SN's public remarks concerning the email and letter sent by TR CO, he appears to conflate a number of facts with those from the letter generated by the TR Medical

---

[311] Email - CJRM – Follow Up to 13 May 20 Phone Call
[312] Email - CJRM – Follow Up to 13 May 20 Phone Call
[313] CNO Ltr Ser 5800 dtd 2 Apr 20
[314] Transcript: DON Press Briefing with Acting Secretary of the Navy Thomas B. Modly and CNO Admiral Gilday dtd 2 Apr 20
[315] Crozier, B. CAPT Statement dtd 15 May 20
[316] How a Ship's Coronavirus Outbreak Became a Moral Crisis for the Military, *NY Times* (6 Apr 20)
[317] Transcript: Acting Navy Secretary Thomas Modly addresses USS Theodore Roosevelt crew about "stupid" ousted captain CNN (6 Apr 20) https://www.cnn.com/2020/04/06/politics/thomas-modly-transcript/index.html

Department. Specifically, in response to a question at his April 2nd press conference, A-SN stated "I think you raise a particular level of alarm when you say that 50 people on the - on the crew are going to die, OK?" This appears to be a reference to a comment in the March 31st letter signed by members of the TR Medical Department in which they conclude that they stood "the potential to have 50 or more fatal cases"[318] aboard TR if their expected case fatality rate remained constant, as the TR CO's March 30th letter makes no such mention of numbers of potential fatalities.[319] Similarly, A-SN stated at the same press conference that the TR CO's email and letter was "sent and copied to a broad array of other people . . . [and] outside of the chain of command."[320] In fact, the email was sent to 10 recipients, all of whom were either in TR's direct operational chain of command (CPF and CCSG-9) or administrative chain of command (CNAP).[321] It did, however, omit C7F, who was in his chain of command. There is no indication from the evidence available during this investigation that TR CO forwarded this letter beyond that initial group. However, the letter from the TR Medical Department was widely distributed via email to a broad array of people from across the Navy medical community by the TR SMO.[322] Of note, SMO's email with a copy of the Medical Department letter was sent to over 160 recipients, all of which were outside the administrative and operational chains of command of TR.

## Resignation of A-SN

Following his remarks aboard TR and subsequent calls for his resignation, including from House Armed Services Committee Chairman Adam Smith (D-WA),[323] A-SN offered his resignation to the Secretary of Defense on April 7, 2020[324] and his resignation was accepted that same day.[325] In his final "Vector" to the Department, A-SN acknowledged his "poor use of words"[326] on the TR and separately offered a public statement "to apologize to the Navy" for his comments to the crew of the TR.[327]

The initial report of the preliminary inquiry into the events surrounding the disembarkation of Sailors from TR in Guam, in response to cases of COVID-19, was

---

[318] Medical Department Letter dtd 31 Mar 20

[319] TR CO Email and Ltr - Request for Assistance in Response to COVID-19 Pandemic dtd 30 Mar 20

[320] Transcript: DON Press Briefing with Acting Secretary of the Navy Thomas B. Modly and CNO Admiral Gilday dtd 2 Apr 20

[321] TR CO Email and Ltr - Request for Assistance in Response to COVID-19 Pandemic dtd 30 Mar 20

[322] Email – TR SMO - Medical Dept Letter dtd 30Mar 20; Email  TR SMO – FWD: Medical Dept Letter dtd 30 Mar 20

[323] Press Release: "Smith Calls for Modly's Removal After Mishandling U.S.S. Theodore Roosevelt COVID-19 Outbreak" dtd 6 Apr 20

[324] A-SN Ltr of 7 Apr 20

[325] SECDEF Ltr of 7 Apr 20

[326] A-SN Ltr of 7 Apr 20 Final Vector SECNAV Final Vector

[327] UPDATED: Modly Resigns Amidst Carrier Roosevelt Controversy; Army Undersecretary to Serve as Acting SECNAV USNI News (7 Apr 20) https://news.usni.org/2020/04/07/modly-offers-resignation-amidst-carrier-roosevelt-controversy

completed on April 7th, prior to the A-SN's resignation. An addendum to the report was provided on April 14th at CNO's request to conduct additional interviews to clarify the timing of conversations between the TR CO and members of his operational and administrative chains of command, as well as whether there were observations of concern during the CSG-9 training cycle prior to deployment. This evaluation revealed that CSG-9 had completed all deployment preparations and certifications with high marks, including having a strong leadership team with disciplined, effective battle rhythm and planning processes.[328]

---

[328] Email (SIPR) - VADM Conn to ADM Burke – "FW: (U) Updated CSG-15 CTX Brief to C3F for 17 December" dtd 13 Apr 20, CSG15 TR C2X Debrief, dtd 20 Dec 19

## Chapter 5 - Opinions and Recommendations

### Summary of Opinions

*The following 18 key opinions were derived from this investigation into the COVID-19 outbreak aboard TR:*

1. ***Based upon the pre-event risk analysis, the decision to execute the Da Nang port visit was appropriate. The visit was executed with sensible precautions, based on the world's understanding of COVID-19 at the time.***

2. ***The former TR CO initially responded appropriately by quarantining 39 Sailors following the Da Nang port visit. However, after three Sailors tested positive for COVID-19 aboard TR on March 24, 2020, the former TR CO failed to put adequate additional measures in place for the rest of the crew to further slow the spread of COVID-19 throughout the ship.***

3. ***The TR SMO's recommendation and the resulting release by the former TR CO of crewmembers in quarantine from the aft portion of the ship on March 29, 2020 likely resulted in infection to a larger portion of the crew.***

4. ***The embarked CSG-9 Warfare Commanders (WCs) (TR CO, CAG CVW-11, DESRON Commodore) and the TR SMO displayed an abundance of concern for the safety of the crew as their primary focus, yet they were unable to develop COAs prior to or even by four days after arrival in Guam that provided for the short-term safety of the crew. Instead, they focused efforts on the most constrained and least executable COA (at the time), while taking insufficient parallel steps that would have resulted in more immediate segregation, quarantine and isolation of the crew. As a result, efforts to move the crew off the ship were uncoordinated, unsupervised and slow. The extended time Sailors remained on the ship, while no longer segregated, likely increased the number of infections.***

5. ***CCSG-9, the embarked CSG-9 WCs, and the former TR CO and TR SMO did not demonstrate effective leadership when they initially took few actions to overcome obstacles to aggressively utilize the approximately 2,300 beds that were made available by Naval Base Guam, likely resulting in infection to a larger portion of the crew.***

6. ***C7F's early focus on the Okinawa option over the Guam hotel option resulted in the TR Strike Group key Captains (CSG-9 COS, former TR CO, TR XO, TR SMO and CVW-11 CAG) believing that C7F did not feel their same sense of urgency for providing proper long term quarantine and isolation quarters. This led these Captains to distrust the C7F staff and hampered their ability to deal with the crisis with the resources that were***

available, or develop alternate courses of action other than the request for 4,000 CDC compliant rooms, which at the time was the most constrained and least likely COA.

7. The former TR CO did not demonstrate forceful backup, effective communication or adequately communicate with his Immediate Superior in Command (CCSG-9, embarked in TR) in that he did not discuss his concern with the lack urgency he perceived from C7F and CCSG-9 on the Guam Hotel option being pursued, prior to sending his letter.

8. CCSG-9 did not provide effective leadership to the former TR CO and the embarked CSG-9 WCs in that he did not effectively address and correct a growing, divisive and counterproductive narrative among his senior officers regarding distrust of C7F or any course of action that did not fit their immediate sense of urgency. Additionally, he did not direct decisive action to ensure prompt execution of the egress of the TR crew. Finally, it is not clear that he effectively advocated for TR's needs to higher headquarters or provided clear feedback to his team when those needs could not meet TR leadership's timeline.

9. The TR SMO developed a flawed, worst-case crew casualty narrative that the CAG CVW-11 reinforced and frequently amplified at Warfare Commander Boards, and that had an impact on the mindset of the former TR CO and TR XO. The TR SMO fostered distrust of HHQ actions, and put his leadership in an untenable situation.

10. The TR CO sent his email and letter as a genuine plea for help from CPF and CNAP. Each leader received and acted upon it as such, responding via phone and email, respectively, within minutes of receipt, with CNAP also ensuring C7F and CJRM were made aware of the request. Further, CPF considered the matter of sending the letter closed after his conversation with both CCSG-9 and TR CO.

11. When asked to sign a letter that contained a flawed, worst-case crew casualty narrative as well as an ultimatum concerning an intent to submit the letter to the public, the TR SMO missed a leadership opportunity to correct subordinates. Instead, he signed the letter, and transmitted it outside the chain of command, essentially endorsing the effort to undermine Navy leadership.

12. The former TR CO intended for his email to be a "red flare" to accelerate needed support and ensure attention to what he believed to be insufficient courses of action. The former TR CO wrote his email to break down communication barriers on plans, resources and support, and did not intend for it to be released to the public. However, he did not personally

*inform his Immediate Superior in Command, CCSG-9, of the letter and instead transmitted information of a very sensitive nature about a capital warship on an unclassified network.*

13. *The exclusion of C7F on the former TR CO's email, as well as the lack of advanced coordination by the former TR CO with CCSG-9 and others, bypassed the operational chain of command and demonstrated poor judgment.*

14. *The former TR CO's email and the attached letter of March 30, 2020 were unnecessary, and had no positive impact on actions already being aggressively pursued by higher headquarters (CJRM, C7F, and CPF).*

15. *Release of the former TR CO's letter to the San Francisco Chronicle complicated the Navy's negotiations with the Government of Guam for use of hotel rooms in Guam.*

16. *Detailed patient history analysis of the 29 personnel received aboard TR via COD following the Da Nang port visit concluded that CODs were not the likely source for the COVID-19 outbreak.  Although the pre-event risk analysis for the Da Nang port visit was assessed as sufficiently thorough and the decision to the execute the port visit was appropriate at the time, the Da Nang port visit was found to be the most likely source of the outbreak on TR.*

17. *Detailed analysis of TR sick call logs revealed that COVID-19 was likely present, yet undetected, as early as March 11, 2020.*

18. *The use of personal protective equipment (PPE) and employment of tactics, techniques, and procedures (TTP) by the TR Medical Department were likely effective, as there was only one COVID-19 infection among TR Medical Department personnel.*

## Recommendations

*The following nine recommendations resulted from this investigation into the COVID-19 outbreak aboard TR:*

1.  **The former TR CO should not be reassigned to command afloat or ashore.**

2.  **Consider appropriate administrative measures for the former TR CO, TR SMO, CAG CVW-11, and CCSG-9. For the TR SMO specifically, a detachment for cause due to substandard performance is recommended.**

3.  **OPNAV perform a study to determine which, if any, coastal states have not been transparent about the number of their COVID-19 cases; port visit approval authorities use the results of the transparency study as an additional factor to weigh when acting upon potential port visits in the future.**

4.  **BUMED coordinate with Naval Warfare Development Command (NWDC) to update to NTRP 4-02.10 in light of the COVID-19 outbreak; OPNAV issue clear requirements concerning minimum precautions and tiered responses for each specific class of ship and submarine that shall occur following potential exposure to a highly transmissible infectious disease.**

5.  **Naval Safety Center lead Cultural Workshops for TR and CSG-9 to identify hazards that result from cultural behaviors associated with poor communication, lack of trust, and integrity.**

6.  **BUMED debrief TR Medical Department to determine what specific personal exposure precautions were taken in the Medical Department and, if appropriate, publish best practices guidance throughout the Navy's medical community and the fleet.**

7.  **Navy leadership use this case study to emphasize the Navy's recent lesson learned from the USS Fitzgerald (DDG 62) and USS John S. McCain (DDG 56) collisions of 2017, in that Navy leaders are willing to listen when commanding officers have concerns about mission readiness or need additional assistance. CPF spoke with CCSG-9 and the TR CO on the phone immediately after the CO's email was sent. In this call, CPF laid out all the actions in progress, and at the end of the conversation, asked CCSG-9 and the TR CO what else they needed. With no additional requests made, CPF considered the matter closed. CPF did not make any notifications up to the CNO/VCNO level until some 30 hours later when it became apparent media had a copy of the letter, and that a story based on the letter, which contained inaccuracies, would soon follow. CNAP's immediate response was "thank you for the red flare... we'll escalate work... immediately."**

*The lessons should also reinforce that although the TR CO's intentions were pure, his method of transmitting his concerns did not display good judgment. Further, the lesson should emphasize some fundamental points if in the position of needing to bypass your immediate superior(s) in command:*

    a. *First, review your actions and check your facts. The Navy's culture prides itself on an open and candid exchange between seniors and subordinates. Look at yourself with a critical eye and make sure you are not missing some key information.*

    b. *Ask yourself why you are there - have you done all you can to communicate your case in clear and unambiguous terms? Just as you would do for a subordinate, you owe that senior an opportunity to correct the situation. Talking to the senior's staff is not a substitute for addressing them directly. A staff representative may not be capable of relaying your case with the detail, rigor or passion that only you can provide.*

    c. *Finally, if you must bypass that senior, recognize this should be considered a last resort. Use a private means of conveying those concerns, such as a phone call or an in-person office call with the next superior, if possible. This allows face-saving opportunities on both sides. The boss's boss may have key information or context that makes you realize you had it wrong.*

8. *CNO, in coordination with 4-star Fleet Commanders, conduct a review of the existing formal course of training for Strike Group Commanders. This review should specifically address the sufficiency of the training curriculum and make recommendations for the mandatory completion of priority training events prior to assumption of Strike Group command. Additionally, this review should make recommendations for the addition of training events focused on developing critical thinking and problem solving during nontraditional operations and unpredictable crisis event response.*

9. *USFFC, in coordination with CPF, propose to CNO how future CSG training and certification events will evaluate the ability of commanders and Strike Group Staffs to deal with "off-script" events in the face of battle, such as the curve-ball thrown by COVID-19. As we go forward, we need Strike Group Commanders, and their supporting staffs, who will not flinch in the face of a distraction like COVID-19 while fully engaged in combat operations.*

**Status of Recommendations from the Preliminary Inquiry**

a. Issue revised Navy-wide COVID-19 guidance to address the magnitude of the problem on TR and strategies for triaging crew members to limited numbers of makeshift quarantine and isolation facilities both aboard the ship and at remote shore locations. **Complete.**

Conduct war games and table-top exercises to optimize various scenarios and conduct shipboard training/exercises. **In progress.**

b. Using the TR case history, develop warship-specific COVID-19 infection spread models. **In progress.**

c. Examine the impact of the ship's decision to release personnel from isolation on March 29th and use this to inform the infection spread model recommended in recommendation b. **In progress.**

d. Examine shipboard and shore-based pre-positioned stores of personal protective equipment, test gear and other equipment necessary to test, diagnose and if necessary ship test samples. **Complete.**

e. Identify key shore nodes for offload of infected crew members with suitable facilities and infrastructure for isolation/quarantine. Institutionalize requirements to assess time/speed/distance to ready nodes versus the delays that may be induced by going to a remote port without adequate facilities. **In progress.**

www.ingramcontent.com/pod-product-compliance
Lightning Source LLC
Chambersburg PA
CBHW050618110426
42813CB00008B/2596